COMPASSION IN NURSING

COMPASSION IN NURSING

THEORY, EVIDENCE AND PRACTICE

EDITED BY ALISTAIR HEWISON AND
YVONNE SAWBRIDGE

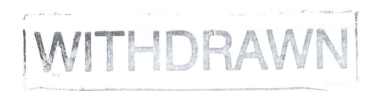

First published 2016 by
PALGRAVE

Palgrave in the UK is an imprint of Macmillan Publishers Limited,
registered in England, company number 785998, of 4 Crinan Street,
London, N1 9XW.

Palgrave Macmillan in the US is a division of St Martin's Press LLC,
175 Fifth Avenue, New York, NY 10010.

Palgrave is a global imprint of the above companies and is represented
throughout the world.

Palgrave® and Macmillan® are registered trademarks in the United States,
the United Kingdom, Europe and other countries.

ISBN 978–1–137–44369–4 paperback

This book is printed on paper suitable for recycling and made from fully
managed and sustained forest sources. Logging, pulping and manufacturing
processes are expected to conform to the environmental regulations of the
country of origin.

A catalogue record for this book is available from the British Library.

A catalog record for this book is available from the Library of Congress.

Printed and bound by CPI Group (UK) Ltd, Croydon, CR0 4YY

CONTENTS

v

LIST OF ILLUSTRATIONS

Figures

Tables

Boxes

Case Studies

ACKNOWLEDGEMENTS

We are grateful to the anonymous reviewers for their helpful comments on an earlier draft of the manuscript. We are also indebted to the team at Palgrave for their support, patience and good humour in helping us produce this book.

The authors and publisher wish to thank the following organisations for kind permission to reproduce copyright material:

Professor Jill Maben, OBE, and the NETSCC (NIHR [National Institute for Health Research] Evaluation, Trials and Studies Coordinating Centre) for Figure 4.1, page 78

The Royal College of Psychiatrists for Figure 5.1: A virtuous circle, page 94

Figure 1.2: Keogh's eight ambitions, page 27, and Figure 1.3: Recommendations of the Berwick Report, page 28, are available through the Open Government License v3.0.

Some of the material in the introduction first appeared in the Journal Recherche et Fomation and is included here with permission. Hewison A & Sawbridge Y (2014). Analysing poor nursing care in hospitals in England: The policy challenge. Recherche et formation, 76, 34–48. ISBN 978-2-84788-758-7. Electronic Reference: Hewison A & Sawbridge Y (2014) Analysing poor nursing care in hospitals in England: The policy challenge. Recherche et Fomation http://rechercheformation.revues.org/2225

FOREWORD

During my long career as a nurse and manager in the National Health Service (NHS), I have, like many people, worked in a system that continually reinforces the importance of compassion as an integral part of the essence of nursing practice. Throughout this time, I have seen first-hand the positive (and lasting) impact nursing has on patients and their families when they feel they have been cared for with compassion, and this has been a great source of professional satisfaction.

However, my experience at Mid Staffordshire NHS Foundation Trust, in the wake of the damning report from the Healthcare Commission in 2009, demonstrated to me the devastating effect on patients and families when they feel 'let down' by the NHS, and particularly when the nursing profession is seen, in their eyes, to have lost sight of its most important professional value: to care with compassion.

This experience has set me on a journey to 'get under the skin' of what constitutes compassionate care, and, crucially, how the system supports the development of a culture that provides staff at the front line of care with the means to deliver it, at each and every contact with the patient.

I was delighted when asked by Yvonne and Alistair to write this foreword, especially as I have been aware of the excellent work they have been leading to generate a more in-depth discussion about compassion in healthcare.

Together with the other contributors to the book, they take the reader through an exploration of the philosophical roots of compassion, analyses of the concept, examination of the policy context, reports from empirical studies investigating compassion in practice and discussion of a number of models/approaches designed to support front-line nurses to deliver compassionate care. Importantly, the creation of a compassionate culture is explored in some detail and is essential reading for those in leadership roles.

The focus for the book was to generate discussion and analysis of a number of key issues in the wake of the narrative depicting a crisis in nursing, and the vilification of individuals and the profession. The development of the 'six Cs' and other initiatives such as values-based recruitment are examples of the system and policy response to failures in care. The contributors to the book seek to give a broader response, stimulate further debate and share knowledge to highlight the complexities and multiple factors affecting the delivery of compassionate care in practice.

Compassion is rarely explored in its full complexity, and this book offers a more in-depth discussion to help nurses and others involved in the delivery and management of healthcare develop a greater understanding of the issues and potential solutions. A major thread running through the book is the increasing importance of the use of human factors science in the development of reliable healthcare systems that recognise the interaction between the individual nurse and the care environment. Too often we set front-line staff up to fail.

This book should be essential reading for all involved in the commissioning of healthcare, leaders, managers (particularly trust boards), policymakers and educators, as well as practising nurses. We all have a primary responsibility to understand the complexities of the delivery of healthcare and to develop a culture which supports and develops our front-line clinical colleagues to deliver safe, high-quality, effective care with compassion.

Although this book draws on a number of perspectives and includes material from contributors with a broad range of relevant expertise, other approaches, of course, have been developed. It is hoped that readers will continue to explore the challenges of delivering compassion in practice, using this book and others as rich sources of evidence to inform the debate.

The challenges for the delivery of healthcare in the future are well documented and understood. This book will help to ensure that the focus on the importance of compassion to patients, their families and of course all those who deliver care, is not lost on the journey.

Sir Stephen Moss
Former Turnaround Chairman,
Mid Staffordshire NHS Foundation Trust,
England
February 2016

CONTRIBUTORS

John Ballatt, *Director, The Openings Consultancy*

John Ballatt offers consultancy to individuals, teams and organisations, mainly in health and social care, often in challenging circumstances. He is a Partner in the multi-disciplinary People in Systems consultancy. He lectures widely on what cultivates and sustains healthy organisational cultures that support staff in giving their best to patients. He is co-author, with Penelope Campling, of 'Intelligent Kindness: reforming the culture of healthcare' (RCPsych 2011).

Before his move to independent work, John's career spanned 30 years in the voluntary, Local Government and NHS sectors. He began work in therapeutic communities, before moving on to train, and then manage social workers, to manage and, for a short time, commission NHS services, with a final six year stint as an Executive Director of a large NHS Trust, with responsibilities for service management and trust-wide Strategic Organisational Change.

Jocelyn Cornwell, *The Point of Care Foundation*

Jocelyn founded The Point of Care programme, originally at The King's Fund in 2007, and went on to become the chief executive of The Point of Care Foundation, an independent charity based in London, in 2013. She originally trained as a medical sociologist and ethnographer and is the author of "Hard-Earned Lives: accounts of health and illness from East London" (1984).

She has worked in academic research, as a senior manager in NHS community health services and in health regulation, first at the Audit Commission and then at the Commission for Health Improvement (CHI) where she was responsible for the design of the national reviews of clinical governance in NHS trusts and eventually acting Chief Executive Officer.

Jocelyn is the external lead for patient and public involvement for the NW London CLARHC, visiting professor in the Department of Medicine at Imperial College London and a trustee of the Nuffield Trust.

Georgina Craig, *National Director, Experience Led Commissioning Programme*

Georgina has over 21 years experience in the health sector. She is passionate about supporting health and care organisations to respond to what matters to people and families. Having worked in healthcare, profit and not for profit sectors in a range of roles during her career, she set up a social enterprise in 2009 to spread and embed innovation in person centred service redesign and commissioning. This filled a gap she saw within NHS systems management thinking which was more focussed on process and efficiency than what mattered to people. Since then, she was worked to develop a novel insights based approach to whole system redesign called Experience Led Commissioning. This process puts what matters to people at the heart of the commissioning process, and generates data from conversations with people and families that provide actionable insights for commissioners and providers – and person centred outcomes and measures that are co-designed locally. Georgina also works at National level, and is a leading member of the National Primary care Network and heads The New NHS Alliance's People Powered Improvement programme, which aims to support primary care to drive improvement in partnership with people and communities.

Marjorie Ghisoni (formerly Lloyd) *Lecturer in Mental Health Nursing, Bangor University*

Marjorie is a mental health nurse lecturer at Bangor University in Wales. Marjorie has worked in pre and post registration nurse education for over 15 years. Previously Marjorie worked as a community psychiatric nurse working closely with service users and their families who have experienced mental illness. Marjorie has studied and worked with third sector organisations to help develop community resources for people who have been disabled by mental illness and in developing coping skills for their recovery. The empowerment and emancipation of people with a mental illness has been a large focus of her work and Marjorie has travelled to the USA and The Netherlands as well as key organisations in Scotland and England to explore evidence based practice. Marjorie has written chapters and books on health care including mental health nursing skills, care planning in health and social care and personalised care planning in mental health care. Marjorie's experience and research has led her towards a strong commitment to teaching and developing compassionate and empowering care in nursing.

Alistair Hewison, *Senior Lecturer, University of Birmingham*

Alistair is Senior Lecturer, and Research Lead for Nursing in the School of Nursing at the University of Birmingham. He worked for many years as a staff nurse, charge nurse and manager in the National Health Service (NHS). His current research and teaching activities are centred on the management and organisation of care, which recently involved the investigations of large scale service re-design in acute hospitals and the organisation of End of Life Care services. Other projects include an evaluation of research capacity in the NHS and examination of staff support systems in nursing. He has an Honorary Contract with Birmingham St Mary's Hospice where he is responsible for research development. International work includes an end of life care research collaboration with colleagues in the School of Nursing at Virginia Commonwealth University, where he also serves as a member of the Advisory Board of the Langston Center for Quality, Safety and Innovation. He has written widely on health care management and policy issues in papers published in scholarly journals and chapters in edited collections.

Valerie Iles, *Really Learning, www.reallylearning.com*

Valerie has spent the last 25 years teaching, writing, and researching about clinical leadership. She offers offer development programmes that enable healthcare professionals and teams to flourish, re-discover their enthusiasm for their roles, enhance their ability to interact effectively with others and encourage them to help their organisations act with care and compassion for patients. Having founded, and served as Director of the Health Management Group at City University, designing and directing three Masters degree programmes, she has continued to work with clinical and management teams across the NHS as a developer, facilitator and mentor. She is an Honorary Professor at the London School of Hygiene and Tropical Medicine and Buckinghamshire New university, and a Fellow of the RCGP. She has written four books and numerous papers published in scholarly journals.

Dr June Jones, *Senior Lecturer, College of Medical and Dental Sciences, University of Birmingham*

June is Senior Lecturer in Biomedical Ethics and College of Medical and Dental Sciences Lead on Religious and Cultural Diversity at the University of Birmingham. She is also the Religion and Health Lead at the Edward Cadbury Centre for the Public Understanding of Religion.

Before her move into academia, June worked as a nurse in Intensive Care. This ignited her desire to understand more about complex ethical decision making and the impact personal beliefs have on the multi-disciplinary team.

Since joining the University in 2000, June has specialised in professional ethics, fostering an inclusive curriculum where respect for equality and diversity is key to realising the success of each student. June was awarded a National Teaching Fellowship from the Higher Education Academy in 2015 in recognition of her work in this area.

Sharon Mastracci, *Associate Professor, University of Utah*

Sharon Mastracci is an Associate Professor in the Department of Political Science and a Fellow in the Hinckley Institute of Politics at the University of Utah. She studies public service employment, and women and gender in public service organizations. Her research on emotional labor with Mary Ellen Guy and Meredith Newman has resulted in numerous publications, including their 2008 book *Emotional Labor: Putting the Service in Public Service.* They are currently studying the effect of culture on the experience of emotional labor in public service work. Sharon was a 2014-2015 Fulbright Scholar to the United Kingdom, and remains an associate at the Institute of Local Government Studies (INLOGOV), University of Birmingham (UK).

Stephen Pattison *is an interdisciplinary scholar with appointments in religion and health care humanities at the Universities of Birmingham, Durham and Glasgow.*

He is a practical theologian and ethicist who studies the relationship between beliefs and values and practices, both within and outside formal 'religions'. One of his principal roles in Birmingham is to direct the Doctor of Practical Theology programme, a part-time degree for researching professionals from a variety of practice backgrounds, religious and other.

Throughout his career Stephen has specialised in the work of chaplaincy in health care, researching how patients and staff relate to beliefs within the health care setting. He has also recorded how chaplaincy has changed in response to multi-cultural needs, and the challenges this raises for chaplaincy education.

Yvonne Sawbridge, *Senior Fellow, Health Services Management Centre*

Yvonne is a Registered General Nurse and Health Visitor by profession, and joined the Health Services Management Centre in May 2011 from her post as a Director of Quality and Executive Nurse in South Staffordshire PCT. She worked in a variety of roles and settings in the NHS over her career, and brings this range of experience with her to her current academic role.

Yvonne designs and delivers a number of leadership programmes, both national and local, and her varied research has included evaluating the National Return to Practice scheme; evaluating the effectiveness of community services, and the effect of the NHS 2012 reforms on Cancer services. However her main research interest focuses on the importance of emotional labour in nursing (and other health and social care professions) as a component of delivering compassionate care to patients and service users. She believes that well cared for staff provide the only route through which all patients can be given the care and compassion they require at their time of need.

Barbara Schofield, *Nurse Consultant for Older People at Calderdale & Huddersfield NHS Foundation Trust*

Barbara is a Nurse Consultant for Older People at Calderdale & Huddersfield NHS Foundation Trust. The Trust has two District General Hospitals and provides some community services. As Nurse Consultant she provides clinical leadership to nurses, and other staff, in the care of older people. Barbara leads on the dementia care strategy for the Trust, and has been involved in numerous national initiatives and groups. She has spent many years developing and applying advanced nursing skills in clinical practice, leadership, management, and service improvement. Throughout this time her passion for 'nursing', that is those qualities patients attribute to what it means to be a 'good nurse', such as empathy, understanding, kindness, and caring for as well as applying care, was reignited. Her job allows her to promote this 'pure' aspect of being a nurse. In 2011, Barbara was awarded the first Claire Rayner Scholarship to undertake a PhD researching Compassion in Nursing. The scholarship has provided a wonderful opportunity to explore what it is to be a good nurse and determine the ways in which this can be encouraged and developed throughout nursing. Her PhD is an exploration of compassion in nursing: the meaning and significance of compassionate nursing care for older people in hospital.

Dr Sonya Wallbank, *Clinical Director of the Arden Centre (www.theardencentre.co.uk)*

Sonya is a Chartered Psychologist and an Associate Fellow of the British Psychological Society (BPS). Sonya is also a registered member of the Health and Care Professional Council (HCPC) and Chartered member of the Chartered Institute of Personnel Development (CIPD).

Sonya is the founder of Capellas Nurseries Group and has worked in the UK, USA and Australia delivering direct therapy and also training a range of staff to utilise her model of restorative resilience within their work. Her most recent NHS position was Director of Children and Families. She has trained a range of staff in the NHS, Department of Health, Local Authorities, private organisations, Hospices and Charities. As a keen writer, Sonya has published in both professional journals and books and has a number of ongoing blogs.

Introduction: The Context of Compassion

Alistair Hewison and Yvonne Sawbridge

Introduction

It has been argued that nursing has been engulfed by a fundamental moral crisis (Phillips, 2011a), which is reflected in a number of observations that have been made about the state of nursing care in hospitals in England of late, and concerns expressed about the decline in the quality of care. Much of the discussion has centred on identifying the causes of this apparent fall in standards. However, although the strident tenor of the debate, much of it conducted through popular media outlets, has highlighted the issue, it has done little to explain the underlying causes or indeed signal a realistic solution. Also, it is a response to a particular set of circumstances and represents only one view. For example, in a recent survey, 86 per cent of the 2002 people interviewed reported nursing to be the most trustworthy profession (Independent, 2015), and others have sought to redress the balance by reporting how the remarkable work of nurses is reflected in the plethora of thank-you cards and other expressions of gratitude they receive (Watson, 2012), and by highlighting the 'joy of nursing' (NHS Greater Glasgow and Clyde, 2015). However, compassion remains a matter of national concern, as reflected in the observation that no one joins the NHS to deliver anything other than exceptional care; [yet] a system has been created that can sometimes make that difficult or even impossible (Department of Health [DH], 2013: 3).

The purpose of this introduction is to explore how and why this has become an issue of national attention in England; to summarise some of the contributory factors by way of explanation of this turn of events; and then to outline the subsequent chapters which analyse different aspects and dimensions of compassion and the approaches being taken to address concerns about care. It will be demonstrated that far from it being a new issue, the latest furore about care is part of a familiar narrative that has charted such failures over a number of years. What is different about the current episode in this tradition, though, is the prominence it has achieved, which in turn has evoked a widespread policy response (see

1

Chapter 1). However, the policy recommendations that have been made are unlikely to be realised without action on a number of fronts, and the final part of this introduction 'sets the scene' by highlighting how the later chapters examine these areas in more detail.

Background

Nurses in England work in a healthcare system which is extremely complex, constantly changing and subject to a high level of external regulation. They have contributed to improvements in quality and the nation's health (NHS England, 2013), and the NHS was recently identified to be the best-performing health system in a comparative analysis of 11 countries (Commonwealth Fund, 2014). Yet despite these clear markers of success, and the existence of an extensive regulatory framework, there have been a number of high-profile reports over the last few years citing shocking cases of poor nursing care. These include the Francis Inquiry (Francis, 2013, 2010); the Health Service Ombudsman's report (Parliamentary and Health Service Ombudsman [PHSO] 2011); Maidstone and Tunbridge Wells (Healthcare Commission, 2007); and the Care Quality Commission report (CQC, 2011). They catalogue a series of failures in the provision of care, such as when patients rang the call bell to summon help from nurses because they were in pain or needed to go to the toilet, it was often not answered, or not answered in time. Families also reported that medication and nutritional supplements were not given on time; some patients were left, sometimes for several hours, in wet or soiled sheets, increasing the risk of infection and pressure sores; and wards, bathrooms and commodes were not always clean (Healthcare Commission, 2009). Elsewhere it was found that difficulties encountered by service users and their relatives were not solely a result of illness, but arose from the dismissive attitude of staff, a disregard for process and procedure, and an apparent indifference of National Health Service (NHS) staff to deplorable standards of care (Parliamentary and Health Service Ombudsman [PHSO], 2011). In addition, although the Care Quality Commission has found many examples of people being treated with respect and receiving personalised, attentive care during its inspections, it also reported that many patients did not receive help with eating and drinking; their care needs were not assessed; and their dignity was not respected (CQC, 2011). The Patients Association (2010) also compiled accounts of poor care which included personal perspectives on the effect this had on the people involved. This resulted in the establishment of a Commission on Dignity in Care (CDC, 2012) which made a series of recommendations and invited responses from individuals and organisations.

These 'official' accounts of poor standards of care have been accompanied by extensive commentary and condemnation in the wider media, which attribute the problems to nurses being educated at too high a level and thus losing sight of caring (Marrin, 2009; Odone, 2011). In addition, the crisis in nursing is seen as part of a far broader and deeper spiritual malaise whereby duty to others and respect for the innate humanity of every person have been eroded by the 'me society' of ruthless, self-centred individualism (Phillips, 2011a).

Shields et al. (2012) regard this as evidence of a cleverly articulated campaign by politicians of all persuasions, and a media which presents a simplistic view of nursing to undermine the notion of university-level education for nurses. Another interpretation is that the current situation bears the hallmarks of a 'moral panic'. Essentially, a moral panic refers to an exaggerated reaction, from the media or wider public, to the activities of particular social groups and an extreme response to a type of behaviour that is seen as a social problem which magnifies the original area of concern (Marsh and Melville, 2011). In this sense, nurses can be regarded as the latest 'folk devils'. This was the term used by Cohen (2011) in his original work investigating the activities of, and reactions to 'mods' and 'rockers'. These were two distinct youth sub-cultures regarded as 'deviant', and Cohen's work was an attempt to offer a sociological explanation of this particular manifestation of delinquency. The attribution of the moral panic label means that the extent and significance of the issue have been exaggerated (i) in itself (compared with other more reliable, valid and objective sources) and/or (ii) compared with other, more serious problems (Cohen, 2011). Although it may seem extreme to characterise the current debate about nursing in these terms, as Cohen (2011) observes, 'Some of the social space once occupied by moral panics has been filled by more inchoate social anxieties, insecurities and fears' (p. xxx).

Justifiable though some of the expressed concerns are, their treatment has served to prevent detailed and constructive debate, because the criticisms levelled at individual 'uncaring' nurses (Odone, 2011; Marrin, 2009), and the discipline as a whole for pursuing a misguided feminist project (Phillips, 2011b), distract attention from the fundamental issues. Indeed, singling nursing out as the main cause of these systemic failures is misleading (Hutchinson, 2015). Even though it is conceded in a more measured later campaign that 'nobody is going to solve the crisis in 1000 words' (Patterson, 2012), the tendency is to sensationalise rather than to analyse the issues. Another factor to consider is that, unfortunately, there is a history of cases of poor care in the NHS. For example in the 1960s and 1970s, the Ely and Normansfield Hospitals were the subject of national inquiries aimed at uncovering the reasons for major lapses in quality (Walshe and Higgins, 2002). However, as is evident from the foregoing discussion, although there have been a number of formal investigations over the years, it is not long before a new case of poor care is exposed in another hospital or care home. This is also an international problem, with service failures occurring in the United States, Australia, New Zealand and Canada as well as the UK (Walshe and Shortell, 2004). This suggests that the 'standard' formulaic response to these scandals is not having the desired effect. However, this tradition continued with the establishment of the Prime Minister's Commission (DH, 2011) and the Nursing and Care Quality Forum (DH, 2012). This in turn has resulted in a surge in policy activity focused on correcting the problems of poor care and lack of compassion (see Chapter 1).

The aim of this introduction is to examine the contributory factors identified in the literature in a little more depth and to argue that it is important to make sense of the complex mix of issues that need to be addressed if compassion in nursing care is to be understood. Without this, irrespective of how many recommendations are made, change will not occur; greater understanding of the issues involved is needed. With this in mind, some of these key areas are examined below, followed by a summary of the later chapters, which extend the discussion further.

Hospital Design – Ward Layout

In seeking to understand why compassion has become a high-profile issue in healthcare, it is necessary to take a range of factors into account. For example there have been a number of major capital redevelopment projects in England in the last few years, which in turn have directed attention to the issue of hospital design (Gesler et al., 2004). The traditional design for hospitals was a number of single-sex, multi-bedded wards known as 'Nightingale wards'. A nursing station was generally situated at the top or middle of the ward, and the patients identified as being the most ill were placed as close as possible to the nursing station to ensure the nurses were able to observe them closely and frequently. A benefit of these wards was that the nurses could see, and be seen, by all the patients. However, hospitals are now designed with different ward layouts because evidence indicates that single-bedded rooms are beneficial as they help reduce the incidence of hospital-acquired infections, improve patient confidentiality and privacy, and are quieter for patients (Ulrich, 2004). Although some dispute this evidence (van de Glind et al., 2007, for example), the challenge has not been sufficient to halt the adoption of this new design. Hospitals incorporating four-bedded bays with bathrooms and toilets, and single en suite rooms, are replacing the Nightingale layout, and the overall intention driving this trend is a desire to improve privacy and dignity for patients and make the environment more therapeutic. However, this design has implications for practice. For example the lack of visibility of nurses working in this configuration of accommodation has led to a need to modify practice in order that purposeful, regular contact with patients is planned, rather than naturally occurring as in the past, to prevent them feeling isolated and neglected. This has taken the form of 'intentional rounding', which originated in the United States, where it has had a positive impact on patients and staff (Meade et al., 2006), and has now been adopted in a number of hospitals in the UK as 'care rounds' and 'comfort' rounds (Studer Group, 2006).

Another consequence of this new hospital design is that patients are now cared for in mixed-sex wards – albeit single-sex bays in the main. Patient concerns about this situation eventually led to a policy directive being issued to reduce mixed-sex accommodation, which was then reinforced in the Operating Framework, which set targets to eliminate mixed-sex accommodation in Trusts (DH, 2010). This target would not have been necessary in the days of 30-bedded, single-sex Nightingale wards, and serves to illustrate how hospital design (as with other management and policy decisions) can have unintended and unwelcome outcomes, in particular contributing to a perception that nurses do not spend enough time with the patients.

Nursing Staff Numbers

It would seem to be self-evident that if patients are to be cared for with compassion, there need to be enough staff to provide it. Yet how many staff is enough? Although evidence exists which suggests that higher nurse staffing levels are positively associated with safer patient care, this does not mean there is a causal relationship between the two (Griffiths et al., 2014; Kane et al., 2007). Consequently, decisions about what is the 'right' number of staff for a shift are difficult to make because patient needs vary depending on their age, condition and a range of other factors. Also, the number of staff required is dependent on their level of skill, expertise and training. Furthermore, the contribution of other disciplines and the way 'safe care' is defined indicate that it is a more complex issue than simply identifying the number of staff. There need to be an appropriate number of staff given the nature of the patients being cared for, the skill mix and educational level of the staff, and clear agreement about what staff are to achieve. Yet the associations between education and staffing numbers suggest that patients in hospitals in which 60 per cent of the nurses had bachelor's degrees, caring for an average of six patients, would have 30 per cent lower mortality than patients in hospitals where only 30 per cent of the nurses had bachelor's degrees, and nurses cared for an average of eight patients (Ball et al., 2012). In addition, an increase of one patient per nurse was associated with a 7 per cent increase in the likelihood of a patient dying within 30 days of admission. Similarly, each 10 per cent increase in the number of nurses with a bachelor's degree was associated with a 7 per cent decrease in this likelihood (Ball et al., 2012). Also, if staffing numbers are insufficient, important nursing tasks, including comforting and talking with patients, educating patients and developing or updating nursing care plans/care, are not completed (Ball et al., 2014). This clearly indicates that staffing levels are crucial if compassionate care is to be provided and that the complex nature of the relationship between staffing and care needs to be appreciated.

Ward/Nurse Leadership

The role of the ward sister/charge nurse is acknowledged as 'the linchpin of healthcare services' (Cole, 2010: 6). The report *Breaking Down Barriers, Driving Up Standards* (Royal College of Nursing [RCN], 2009) collated the findings from both the literature and a number of focus groups held with over 90 ward sisters. It identified three key components of the role, which involves being a

1. clinical nursing expert;
2. manager and leader of the ward staff team and the ward environment; and
3. educator (of nursing and nurses, other healthcare professionals, patients and carers).

However, it was found that the role is often poorly defined and inadequately supported and that there are tensions between being perceived as the clinical expert by nurses and doctors, and ward managers by healthcare managers:

> Ward sisters viewed their management work as one component of their role alongside clinical expertise, leadership and teaching, but perceived health care managers to view them *primarily* as managers of staff and ward resources. (RCN, 2009: 6)

Westmoreland (1993) revealed the isolation and loneliness experienced by ward managers as they struggled to balance what they regarded as two competing paradigms of healthcare (which she characterised as being dominated by nursing concerns about the patient/carer on one hand and management/economic priorities on the other). In addition to these tensions, the RCN report highlighted their role in delivering on key performance measures such as waiting times, which were of significant importance to the organisation and therefore needed to be prioritised, but diverted time and attention away from the three core components of their role identified above. These pressures are played out at ward level and affect the environment of care. For example, Thomas (2006) used systems theory to describe how organisational factors can affect staff. She describes a scenario in which a manager becomes frustrated because of an inability to meet unrealistic targets, which results in anger borne of this frustration being transmitted to staff in the department, culminating in the receptionist being unhelpful to a patient. When the ward leader is prevented from showing compassion for his or her staff, it becomes clear how the staff team in turn may have less capacity for providing care in a compassionate manner. The change from ward sister/charge nurse to the commonly used title of 'ward manager' adds further dissonance concerning whether the prime purpose of the role is clinical leadership or ward management. It was noted in the RCN study (RCN, 2009) that the ward sisters/charge nurses unanimously rejected the title 'ward manager' as they had taken on the role in order to 'manage their ward and ward team by a passion for nursing, rather than an aspiration or desire to be "a manager" per se' (p. 6). Their aspiration was to be the lead nurse in charge of the ward, and their identity as a nurse was crucial because this enabled them to lead, with a focus on improving patient care. Their frustrations lay in dealing with staff management issues, budget responsibilities and a variety of other roles which impeded their capacity to find time to be the clinical leader.

It seems that despite the wealth of evidence collated over a number of years which reinforces the importance of the ward sister/charge nurse role (Ogier, 1982; Orton, 2001; Pembrey, 1980), the recommendations from the RCN and other reviews have not been extensively adopted in practice. These findings have been confirmed by the international evidence, which has demonstrated that relationship or people-focused leadership contributes to improving outcomes for the nursing workforce and increases productivity and effectiveness (Cummings et al., 2010). The conclusion of this systematic review was that energy should be invested in building relationships with nurses and that relational leaders positively affect the health and well-being of the nurses in their teams, and, ultimately, the outcomes for patients (Cummings et al., 2010). Similarly, Laschinger, Finegan and Wilk (2011) found that empowering work environments were the result of positive relationships between nurses and their unit managers and promoted job satisfaction. This requires a three-dimensional model of leadership, incorporating attention to relationships, processes and culture, which creates the prerequisites for good patient care during periods of change and in everyday practice (Salmela, Erikkson and Fagerström, 2012). This may suggest that senior managers, policymakers and indeed the public may have difficulty recognising that the leadership of nursing – both at ward and board level – is a full-time occupation in its own right. McKenna et al. (2006) proffer an explanation, stating:

> Many people feel that nursing is common sense, a trait with which you are born, that the caring woman next door can do it expertly and that kindness, respect and compassion are the main criteria for becoming a nurse. (McKenna et al., 2006: 135)

Although these qualities are important, McKenna et al. argue that being a registered nurse involves much more than being kind, because they are accountable for the care of patients who have a myriad of complex health and social care needs. Patients present from varied cultural backgrounds, with increasing expectations of individualised care being provided for them as partners and consumers of healthcare rather than passive recipients. If this is not recognised, and nursing is viewed as a simple task, then the leadership requirements will also be seen as undemanding, which may explain why nurse leadership roles do not have a singular focus on nursing. It would also explain why the current debate is focusing on unidimensional issues – such as individual behaviour or educational changes alone – rather than the wider determinants of practice highlighted in the literature.

A picture emerges, then, that the roles and responsibilities of nurse leaders are multifaceted in the English NHS, and this can lead to their focus being diverted away from professional practice, standards and the development of nursing, towards organisational management concerns and targets. It has also been found that only 10 per cent of junior nurses interested in career progression aspire to being a ward sister/charge nurse (Wise, 2007). The reasons given included lack of direct patient contact, significant workload pressures, long hours and poor pay (Wise, 2007). Although the ward sister/charge nurse job description matches Band 7 in the national framework for pay (Agenda for Change), the RCN (2009) found many ward sisters/charge nurses were paid at Band 6. Other Band 6 roles in the NHS include information technology (IT) trainer, and procurement negotiator – neither of which have the levels of responsibility for patient care or the unsocial hours associated with some ward sister/charge nurse posts.

It is evident then that the role widely considered to be the most important in hospital nursing care is not always adequately supported by the system to enable delivery of its prime focus on clinical care, nor is it sufficiently remunerated or rewarded at a level which encourages others to take it on. This situation can contribute to an environment in which compassionate care is difficult to deliver.

Targets

Considerable discussion has taken place concerning the effect of performance targets on behaviour in healthcare organisations. The Health and Safety Executive (2001) described the importance of measurement in developing the right environment for safety, summarising this approach by citing Drucker (1993), who maintained, 'You can't manage what you can't measure.' The King's Fund (2010) conducted a literature review to assess how the NHS had progressed in terms of a number of performance measures and found that it had been largely successful in meeting the Government's targets and that this indicated an improvement in patient care, for example reducing waiting times from 18 months to 18 weeks for critical operations such as coronary artery bypass surgery. However, it also summarised some of the 'problems' with targets, particularly with regard to how they can affect behaviour and divert attention away from clinical concerns. These included the rush to admit patients to inpatient beds to ensure patients treated in the accident and emergency (A&E) department were there for no longer than four hours. It has been reported that in the ten minutes prior to the expiry of the maximum four-hour wait period, a target set by the last Labour Government, 66 per cent of patients were admitted from A&E, which is 21 per cent of the total number of patients who pass through the A&E department (King's Fund, 2010). This 'last-minute' rush to meet the deadline results in patients being moved at short notice and pressure on staff to complete their work quickly. With regard to the general waiting time target, it was found in a survey of consultants in eight NHS trusts that a 'significant minority' of them felt attempts to meet maximum waiting-time targets clashed with their own clinical judgements concerning when to admit patients from waiting lists, although no evidence was found of substitution of lesser for more serious cases (King's Fund, 2005). This can have serious consequences such as at the Mid Staffordshire NHS Foundation Trust, where it was reported that an over-reliance on process measures and targets was at the expense of focusing on the quality of services provided to patients (Francis, 2013; Colin-Thomé, 2009). Targets can also result in the concentration of resources in one area at the expense of others of equal importance. Infection control targets, for example, have been met but apply to a limited range of infections and at-risk populations (Millar, 2009). Although efforts to deal with methicillin-resistant *Staphylococcus aureus* (MRSA) have been the focus of media attention, being the first healthcare-acquired infection (HAI) for which a target was set, it accounts for only 2 per cent of HAIs in the NHS as a whole (Millar, 2009).

However, as both Bevan and Hood (2006) and the King's Fund report (2010) found, the focus on targets can have an undesirable effect on behaviour. Effectively, what begins to happen is that the focus shifts to the delivery of quantitative targets. This creates difficulties for nurses, as their prime function is to deliver compassionate care, which can be difficult to describe and measure in quantitative terms. Clearly, performance targets can help improve services, particularly in relation to waiting times; however, they can lead to unintended consequences, including the distortion of clinical priorities and the neglect of other non-targeted activities which are equally important, such as time spent with patients. This may be more an outcome of how the targets were implemented and enforced rather than a fault with targets as a whole (King's Fund, 2010), yet it helps explain how an environment can become less patient centred.

Organisational Culture

The importance of culture in determining the way organisations function has attracted a great deal of interest since the 1980s, when the pioneering work of Peters and Waterman (1982) brought its importance to prominence. They argued that if the organisational culture was 'right', excellent performance would result. This continues to be a key concern for management (Collins, 1998), and it has been the focus of extensive empirical study in the English NHS, where the links between culture and quality care are of concern. For example in a comprehensive examination of organisational culture in the NHS, Mannion et al. (2010) concluded that culture matters in terms of 'high levels of quality and performance in NHS' (p. 217). However, it is very complex, defies 'simple categorization and is context dependent' (p. 217). Also, in a study examining the links between organisational culture and patient safety, McKee et al. (2010) found that the value attached to patient safety and staff well-being by senior staff – and particularly by the chief executive – is important in galvanising the organisation and that leadership is important. It is beyond the scope of this introduction to examine the vast amount of literature which addresses organisational culture in healthcare (see Mannion et al., 2005, and Scott et al., 2003, for helpful reviews). Nevertheless, it is important to note the influence of culture on the way nurses deliver care, as this is a crucial determinant of quality.

A number of studies have identified what is required if a supportive organisational culture is to be created. For example the Boorman review (DH, 2009) identified the economic costs of staff stress and called on Trusts to implement staff well-being strategies. An example of these principles being implemented successfully can be found in the United States in the work of Aiken et al. (2000), who identified 'Magnet hospitals', which are organisations that attend to important human factors including staffing levels, engagement and autonomy, enabling them to attract and retain committed nurses. This then becomes a virtuous circle, improving mortality and morbidity outcomes for patients. They concluded:

> Magnet hospitals work. The American Nurses Credentialing Center recognized Magnet Hospitals nurses had lower burnout rates and higher levels of job satisfaction and gave the quality of care provided at their hospitals' higher ratings ... Our findings validate the ability of the Magnet Nursing Services Recognition Program to successfully identify hospitals that provide high quality care. (Aiken et al., 2000: 31)

Similarly, reference to culture has become a familiar theme in policy in this area, with frequent calls for culture change (Francis, 2013; Berwick, 2014). This follows earlier recommendations made in the *Organisation with a Memory* report (DH, 2000), indicating that awareness of the importance of culture and its impact on care has been recognised for many years. More recently, the chief nursing officer in the DH published a framework for best practice entitled *Confidence in Caring* (DH, 2008), which identified how nurses could use the following five 'Confidence creators' to shape a culture in which patients felt secure:

➢ A calm, clean, safe environment.

➢ A positive, friendly culture.

➢ Well-managed care with efficient delivery.

➢ Personalised care for and about every patient.

➢ Good team working and good relationships.

This appears to be a simple checklist to follow, yet determining its impact on practice is difficult. This resonates with the findings from the inquiries noted earlier (Walshe and Higgins, 2002), in that making even small changes in a system as complex and unwieldy as the NHS can be an exacting challenge and often proves unachievable. However, this should not detract from efforts to make the changes in the culture necessary to create an environment where compassionate care is central.

Cultures of engagement, positivity, caring, compassion and respect for all – staff, patients and the public – provide the ideal environment within which to care for the health of the nation. When we care for staff, they can fulfil their calling of providing outstanding professional care for patients. (West and Dawson, 2011: 7)

This concept of looking after staff is not new and is the basis of all good management practice. It involves engaging staff more directly in key decisions about the way care is organised (Ham, 2014; West and Dawson, 2012), and Aiken et al.'s work (2000) demonstrates that where effort is concentrated on creating the right work environment for staff, improvements in patient care result. The current debate in England, which apportions blame to nurses and their education for organisational failures, does not take account of these findings. However, the evidence is clear on the importance of creating cultures in which the key thing that matters and is measured is compassionate care, and when nurses are supported and good leadership is evident at all levels in the organisation, high-quality compassionate care is delivered.

Pre-registration Nurse Education

Another area which has attracted a good deal of attention is pre-registration nurse education. There has been considerable debate in the medical (Delamonthe, 2011) and popular press (Templeton, 2004) about pre-registration nurse education failing to produce nurses who are able to deliver compassionate care. The history of formal and regulated nurse training is generally considered to have begun with the Nightingale Model (Baly, 1997), which was developed in nurse training schools housed in individual hospitals. Student nurses stayed largely within the hospital setting throughout their training and had classroom-based tutorials covering nursing theory, anatomy and physiology, pathology, pharmacology and so on, provided by nurse tutors. These tutors also visited the students on their wards and assessed their practice as part of the formal requirements of the programme. Student nurses were, in effect, apprentices and worked on the wards and departments as part of the nursing staffing establishment (Moores and Moult, 1979). Although the emphasis on the apprenticeship model of nurse training is regarded by some as beneficial, it also resulted in junior nursing students being in charge of wards on night shifts without the requisite experience to provide safe care, because they were included in the rostered staff complement. This system was criticised for its exploitative nature in using students as part of the workforce, and the need for change was identified because of concerns that young women, the traditional pool of entrants for nurse training, had many more attractive employment and education opportunities, which were having an adverse effect on student recruitment (Menzies, 1960; Benner and Wrubel, 1989; United Kingdom Central Council for Nursing, Midwifery and Health Visiting [UKCC], 1986). In response, Project 2000 was introduced, leading to major changes in the way student nurses were trained (UKCC, 1986). The purpose of these reforms was to produce 'knowledgeable doers' and to teach nurses 'how to learn and how to analyse and to provide them with the confidence and motivation to develop themselves in a changing environment' (UKCC, 1985). A diploma qualification, studied at universities, replaced the certificate that had been awarded by the nursing schools, and nursing students were supernumerary during practice placements (often misconstrued as 'observation only'). So rather than being in 'school' for 30 weeks out of the total 156 of their training, nurses now spent 40 per cent of their time at university and 60 per cent in practice (Smith, 2012). This was later adjusted to a 50/50 ratio equating to 2300 hours theory and 2300 hours practice (Nursing and Midwifery Council [NMC], 2004; UKCC, 1999). The number of students completing their programmes under both schemes was, and remains, an issue of concern. Menzies identified this as long ago as 1960, and current attrition rates range from 6 to 20 per cent across institutions (Waters, 2008), reaching 30 per cent in some places (Smith, 2012), even though education providers are penalised if attrition exceeds 13 per cent (DH, 2009b). Although universities are subject to performance management to reduce attrition, many of the causes of students leaving programmes are outside of the control of universities, for example the discrepancy between expectation and reality of practice on the part of students, and stress (Orton, 2011). These are part of the wider educational experience of students, involving balancing studying and working, and the pressures inherent in the clinical environment (see below).

Despite this enduring problem, there is evidence which links higher education with improved outcomes for patients. McKenna et al. (2006) argue that to meet present and future health and social care challenges, nurses must be analytical, assertive, creative, competent, confident, computer literate, decisive, reflective, embracers of change, critical doers and consumers of research, and that these qualities were not inculcated in the old apprenticeship system of nurse training (p. 135). Similarly, Maben and Griffiths (2008) found there is no objective evidence to support the anecdotal view held by some that educating nurses is linked to the 'loss' of caring from the heart of the profession. Furthermore, the evidence from research demonstrates a strong association between the number of staff employed in hospitals who are degree educated and lower patient mortality rates (Aiken et al., 2014). Although data on nurses' qualifications are not held centrally, around 30 per cent of nurses in the UK are estimated to have a degree (Gough and Masterson, 2010). In October 2008, the NMC took the decision to bring England in line with the rest of the UK nurse education system, and the minimum academic level for pre-registration nursing education is now at degree level (NMC, 2011). This development has been greeted with admiration in the United States by campaigners seeking to increase the number of nurses trained at the baccalaureate level from the current level of 50 to 80 per cent of the workforce by 2020 in order to meet the healthcare needs of an ageing population (Institute of Medicine, 2010). However, it continues to be identified as a contributory issue in the provision of poor care, despite evidence to the contrary.

Summary

The purpose of this introduction was to demonstrate that poor care is the result of a combination of factors. Attributing it to single causes such as 'uncaring nurses' or 'the education system' is simplistic and unhelpful. It is important to recognise that if the complex mix of issues that contribute to poor care is to be addressed, then action is required in a number of areas which need to be examined in more detail if they are to be better understood. For example the changes to the physical environment of the acute ward, which have had a negative impact on caring in some settings, can be ameliorated by the introduction of 'intentional rounding', which has the potential to overcome the constraints of the new environments and enable nurses to improve the care they provide for patients. However, caution is required with regard to how it is introduced. The benefits lie in the way nurses interact with patients, not just completing a tick-box form to record that a round has been carried out. This requires a wider set of cultural influences and role modelling, which underpin the introduction of the system.

Central to this is the role of the ward sister/leader. The erosion of the clinical and ward leadership role of the ward sister/charge nurse (RCN, 2009) has resulted in the leadership of care becoming diffuse. Recent policy reviews (DH, 2010, 2011) have advocated that the leadership role of the ward sister/manager be strengthened. It was recognised that the leadership exhibited by ward sisters and charge nurses is pivotal and that it has an unambiguous link to the quality of care and the reputation of the profession. However, ward sisters/charge nurses must be given time to lead, and that time devoted to bureaucratic tasks must be reduced, so they have time to supervise staff and the delivery of care (DH, 2011). Indeed, the Nursing and Care Quality Commission, established at the request of the prime minister, identified that strong, empowered and accountable nurse leadership is crucial to the delivery of safe, compassionate, high-quality care and to the motivation and satisfaction of staff who provide the care. Furthermore, having a leader whose role is focused on organising and co-ordinating the ward; supervising and supporting staff; spending time talking to people in their care, and their loved ones; and ensuring standards are maintained will build good team dynamics and achieve positive care outcomes (DH, 2012). In order to achieve this, it is recommended that ward sisters be made supernumerary so that they have the time to lead; their authority over all matters of ward organisation is reinstated; and they are provided with leadership development support to enable them to lead care (DH, 2012).

These measures will need to be underpinned by a fundamental change in culture so that, as well as ensuring government targets are achieved, a focus is maintained on the importance of care. Strengthening the role of the ward sister will help to some extent; however, action at Board level is also required (Burdett Trust for Nursing, 2010, 2006). In the early days of targets and the developing performance regime in the NHS, there was little that related to outcomes for patients or focused on nursing care specifically. To redress this and ensure that nursing can also be measured, managed and improved, 'clinical dashboards', informed by work such as that conducted by the National Nursing Research Unit (Griffiths et al., 2008), have been developed to capture a range of nursing metrics, such as falls assessment and nutrition and patient experience measures. Their use can help build a culture in which nursing care is seen as central and equally important as economic and other numerical targets. Central to the delivery of the service and the provision of compassionate care is adequate staffing. Evidence demonstrates that the quality of care deteriorates when the ratio of nursing staff to patients falls (Rafferty et al., 2007; Aiken et al., 2010). Other factors are involved, as noted earlier; however, if healthcare organisations are to provide care for patients that improves outcomes and is compassionate, then sufficient numbers of appropriately educated nursing staff are needed.

The Structure of the Book

Ward design, staff numbers, nurse leadership, nurse education and organisational culture are just five of the factors that affect the extent to which compassionate care can be delivered. If nurses are to be able to deliver compassionate care, then a number of issues have to be considered. In the remainder of the book, a range of contributors examine these issues in more detail. The four chapters in Section 1 explore the different ways compassion can be defined and understood. Chapter 1 approaches this from a policy perspective and examines recent policy documents to determine how compassion is interpreted as an activity by the DH and other influential individuals and organisations. This is followed in Chapter 2 by an analysis of the historical roots of the concept of compassion, particularly in the Judaeo/Christian religious tradition, and the implications of this for contemporary practice. This is important because current debates can be clouded by moralistic overtones of duty and 'goodness', at the expense of consideration of wider structural forces affecting practice. The analysis is extended in Chapter 3 to encompass a broader range of components of the concept which set it in a more contemporary nursing context. The final chapter in this section, Chapter 4, explores patients' perspectives of compassion. The combination of the material presented in this first section is intended to clarify the nature of compassion and demonstrate that it is complex, and thus, when defined as a 'problem', is not amenable to simplistic solutions.

In Section 2, the processes involved in delivering compassionate care are discussed. In Chapter 5, the relationship between kindness and compassion will be explored to illustrate what motivates and assures compassionate practice. The need for those working in healthcare to develop 'intelligent kindness' is advocated as part of a wider organisational change that needs to occur if compassion is to be at the heart of care. Drawing on a programme of work conducted to investigate compassion in practice, Chapter 6 examines the evidence for the benefits of a compassionate approach to care. The developing evidence base for the benefits of compassion is evaluated to demonstrate that not only is it good for patients, but it is good for organisations as a whole too. The concluding chapter of this section, Chapter 7, reports a comprehensive programme of work undertaken by the King's Fund to put compassion back into care.

Section 3 is made up of four chapters which consider some of the wider management and organisational challenges involved in delivering compassionate care. First, Chapter 8 argues that unless nurses are supported to meet the emotional demands of their work, it is very difficult for them to demonstrate genuine compassion. Chapter 9 presents a critique of the organisational elements of the health system that have contributed to some of the current difficulties with regard to delivering compassionate care. Clear recommendations for the change needed to address these difficulties are also included. A particular approach to supporting staff and enabling them to care is reported in Chapter 10. Restorative supervision can help practitioners manage the demands made on them more effectively and so help ensure they can continue to provide compassionate care in the face of increasing work pressures. Finally, Chapter 11, provides an international perspective and demonstrates that other health and public sector workers experience problems in trying to care with compassion. The conclusion draws together the themes developed in the book as a whole and suggests that compassionate care can be, and in many instances is being, provided. However, if it is to become the 'norm', then the issues identified in the chapters will have to be addressed.

Each chapter takes a different approach to the material presented. This includes the presentation of detailed empirical findings from PhD studies and other research projects, reports of programmes of work to support compassionate practice, and wide-ranging analyses of the policy and organisational components of compassion. The aim is to provide a range of insights on the issues that stimulate thought and encourage further analyses of compassion in nursing.

Conclusion

The delivery of poor nursing care occurs as a result of a combination of factors, some of which have been examined in this introduction. This suggests that if genuine solutions are to be found, then seeking a 'quick', or indeed a single, fix is misguided. However, changing the culture of healthcare to ensure that the importance of care is at the centre of healthcare organisation will take time and sustained action on the part of all healthcare staff. Systems of support for nurses, embedded in organisations, must underpin this effort so that nurses are able to care for others. Action is needed on all these fronts if the policy and professional challenge of eliminating poor care is to be met and progress sustained. The chapters that follow indicate what sort of action is needed and how it can be brought about.

References

Aiken, L. H, D. M. Sloane, L. Bruyneel, K. Van den Heede, P. Griffiths, R. I. Busse et al. (2014) 'Nurse Staffing and Education and Hospital Mortality in Nine European Countries: A Retrospective Observational Study', *The Lancet*, 383(9931), 1824–30.

Aiken, L. H., D. M. Sloane, J. P. Cimiotti, S. P. Clarke, L. Flynn, J. A. Seago et al. (2010) 'Implications of the California Nurse Staffing Mandate for Other States', *Health Services Research*, 45(4), 904–21.

Aiken, L., D. Havens and D. Sloane (2000) 'The Magnet Nursing Services Recognition Program', *The American Journal of Nursing*, 100(3): 26–36.

Ball, J. E., T. Murrells, A. M. Rafferty, E. Morrow and P. Griffiths (2014) '"Care Left Undone" during Nursing Shifts: Associations with Workload and Perceived Quality of Care', *BMJ Quality & Safety*, 23(2), 116–25.

Ball, J., G. Pike, P. Griffiths, A. M. Rafferty and T. Murrells (2012) 'RN4CAST Nurse Survey in England', National Nursing Research Unit, www.safestaffing. org.uk/downloads/rn4cast-nurse-survey-in-england, accessed 27 April 2016.

Benner, P. and J. Wrubel (1989) *The Primacy of Caring; Stress and Coping in Health and Illness* (Menlo Park, CA: Addison-Wesley).

Berwick, D. (2013). *A Promise to Learn – A Commitment to Act* (London: National Advisory Group on Patient Service).

Bevan, G. and C. Hood (2006) 'What's Measured is What Matters: Targets and Gaming in the English Public Healthcare System', *Public Administration*, 84(3): 517–38.

Burdett Trust for Nursing (2010) *Factors Associated with Clinical Focus in NHS Trust Boards* (London: Burdett Trust for Nursing).

Burdett Trust for Nursing (2006) *Who Cares Wins – Leadership and the Business of Caring* (London: Burdett Trust for Nursing).

Care Quality Commission (CQC) (2011) *Dignity and Nutrition Inspection Programme: National Overview* (London: Care Quality Commission).

Cohen, S. (2011) *Folk Devils and Moral Panics – The Creation of the Mods and Rockers* (London: Routledge).

Cole E. (2010) 'Ward Sisters Need More Power, Leadership Summit Told', *Nursing Management*, 17(4): 6.

Colin-Thomé, D. (2009) *Mid Staffordshire NHS Foundation Trust: A Review of Lessons Learnt for Commissioners and Performance Managers Following the Healthcare Commission Investigation*, www.midstaffsinquiry.com/assets/docs/Colin-Thome%20report.pdf, accessed 10 November 2012.

Collins, D. (1998) *Organizational Change: Sociological Perspectives* (London: Routledge).

Commission on Dignity in Care (2012) *Delivering Dignity* (London: Commission on Dignity in Care).

The Commonwealth Fund (2014) 'Mirror Mirror on the Wall – How the Performance of the U.S. Healthcare System Compares Internationally', www.commonwealthfund.org/publications/fund-reports/2014/jun/mirror-mirror, accessed 20 August 2015.

Cummings, G. G., T. MacGregor, M. Davey, H. Lee, C. A. Wong, E. Lo et al. (2010) 'Leadership Styles and Outcome Patterns for the Nursing Workforce and Work Environment: A Systematic Review', *International Journal of Nursing Studies*, 47: 363–85.

Department of Health (DH) (2013) *The Government Response to the House of Commons Health Committee Third Report of Session 2013–14: After Francis: Making a Difference* (London: DH).

Department of Health (DH) (2012) Nursing and Care Quality Commission Letter to the Prime Minister, 18 May, www.dh.gov.uk/health/files/2012/05/NCQF-letter-to-PM.pdf, accessed 25 July 2012.

Department of Health (DH) (2011) *The Government's Response to the Recommendations in Front Line Care: The Report of the Prime Minister's Commission on the Future of Nursing and Midwifery in England*, www.gov.uk/government/uploads/system/uploads/attachment_data/file/215665/dh_125985.pdf, accessed 27 April 2016.

Department of Health (DH) (2010) *Front Line Care: The Future of Nursing and Midwifery in England. Report of the Prime Minister's Commission on the Future of Nursing and Midwifery in England 2010* (London: DH).

http://webarchive.nationalarchives.gov.uk/20100331110400/http://cnm. independent.gov.uk/wp-content/uploads/2010/03/front_line_care.pdf, accessed 6 May 2011.

Department of Health (DH) (2009a) *NHS Health and Well Being: Final Report* (London, The Stationery Office).

Department of Health (2009b) *Education Commissioning for Quality* (London: The Stationery Office).

Department of Health (DH) (2008) *Confidence in Caring: A Framework for Best Practice* (London: The Stationery Office).

Department of Health (2000) *Organisation with a Memory: Report of an Expert Group on Learning from Adverse Events in the NHS* (London, The Stationery Office).

Drucker, P. (1993) *Managing for Results* (New York: Harper Business).

Francis, R. (2013) *Report of the Mid Staffordshire NHS Foundation Trust Public Inquiry*, www.gov.uk/government/uploads/system/uploads/attachment_data/file/279124/0947.pdf, accessed 21 August 2015.

Francis, R. (2010) *Independent Inquiry into Care Provided by Mid Staffordshire January 2005–March 2009* (London: The Stationery Office).

Gesler, W., M. Bell, S. Curtis, P. Hubbard and S. Francis (2004) 'Therapy by Design: Evaluating the UK Hospital Building Program', *Health Place*, 10(2): 117–28.

Gough, P. and A. Masterson (2010) 'A Mandatory Graduate Entry to Nursing', *British Medical Journal*, 341: c3591.

Griffiths, P., J. Ball, J. Drennan, L. James, J. Jones, A. Recio-Saucedo et al. (2014) 'The Association between Patient Safety Outcomes and Nurse/Healthcare Assistant Skill Mix and Staffing Levels and Factors That May Influence Staffing Requirements', www.nice.org.uk/guidance/sg1/documents/safe-staffing-guideline-consultation5.

Griffiths P., S. Jones, J. Maben and T. Murrells (2008) *State of the Art Metrics for Nursing: A Rapid Appraisal* (London: Kings College).

Ham, C. (2014) *Improving NHS Care by Engaging Staff and Devolving Decision Making. Report of the Review of Staff Engagement and Empowerment in the NHS* (London: King's Fund).

Health and Safety Executive (2001) *A Guide to Measuring Health and Safety Performance*, www.hse.gov.uk/opsunit/index.htm, accessed 5 September 2011.

Healthcare Commission (2009) *Investigation into Mid Staffordshire NHS Foundation Trust* (London: Commission for Healthcare Audit and Inspection).

Healthcare Commission (2007) *Investigation into Outbreaks of Clostridium difficile at Maidstone and Tunbridge Wells* (London: Healthcare Commission).

Hutchinson, J. S. (2015) 'Scandals in Health-Care: Their Impact on Health Policy and Nursing', *Nursing Inquiry*. doi: 10.1111/nin.12115, 1–10.

Independent (2015) 'These Are the 12 Most and Least Trusted Professions in Britain', Indy 100 Independent, http://i100.independent.co.uk/article/these-are-the-12-most-and-least-trusted-professions-in-britain--bJWXJhZKEe, accessed 20 August 2015.

Institute of Medicine (2010) The Future of Nursing: Leading Change, Advancing Health, USA, Robert Wood Johnson Foundation, www.iom.edu/Reports/2010/The-Future-of-Nursing-Leading-Change-Advancing-Health.aspx, accessed 6 October 2011.

Kane, R. L., T. A. Shamliyan, C. Mueller, S. Duval and T. J. Wilt (2007) 'The Association of Registered Nurse Staffing Levels and Patient Outcomes: Systematic Review and Meta-analysis', *Medical Care*, 45(12), 1195–1204.

Laschinger, H.K.S., J. Finegan and P. Wilk (2011) 'Situational and Dispositional Influences on Nurses' Workplace Well-Being: The Role of Empowering Unit Leadership', *Nursing Research*, 60(2), 124–31.

Maben, J. and P. Griffiths (2008) *Nurses in Society: Starting the Debate* (London: Kings College).

Mannion, R., H. Davies, S. Harrison, F. Konteh, R. Jacobs, R. Fulop et al. (2010) *Changing Management Culture and Organisational Performance in the NHS* (London: National Institute for Health Research Service Delivery and Organisation Programme).

Mannion, R., H. Davies and M. Marshall (2005) 'Cultural Attributes of "High" and "Low" Performing Hospitals', *Journal of Health Organization and Management*, 19(6): 431–9.

Marrin, M. (2009) 'Fallen Angels: The Nightmare Nurses Protected by Silence', www.timesonline.co.uk/tol/comment/columnists/minette_marrin/article6814962.ece, accessed 12 October 2011.

Marsh, I. and G. Melville (2011) 'Moral Panics and the British Media – A Look at Some Contemporary "Folk Devils"', *Internet Journal of Criminology*, 2045–6743, 1–21.

McKee, L. (2010) *Understanding the Dynamics of Organisational Culture Change: Creating Safe Places for Patients and Staff* (London: NHIR SDO Programme).

McKenna, H., D. Thompson, R. Watson and I. Norman (2006) 'The Good Old Days of Nurse Training: Rose Tinted or Jaundiced View?', *International Journal of Nursing Studies*, 43: 135–7.

Meade C., A. Bursell and L. Ketelsen (2006) 'Effects of Nursing Rounds on Patients' Call Light Use, Satisfaction and Safety', *American Journal of Nursing*, 106(9): 58–70.

Menzies, I.E.P. (1960) 'A Case-Study in the Functioning of Social Systems as a Defence against Anxiety: A Report on a Study of the Nursing Service of a General Hospital', *Human Relations*, 13(2): 95–121.

Millar, M. (2009) 'Do We Need an Ethical Framework for Hospital Infection Control?', *Journal of Hospital Infections*, 73(3): 232–38.

Moores, B. and A. Moult (1979) 'Patterns of Nurse Activity', *Journal of Advanced Nursing*, 4: 137–49.

NHS England (2013) *A Call to Action – The NHS Belongs to the People* (London: NHS England).

NHS Greater Glasgow and Clyde (2015) 'Joy of Nursing', www.nhsggc.org.uk/our-performance/celebrating-nurses-midwives/history-and-traditions-of-nursing/a-nurses-30-year-story/joy-of-nursing/, accessed 20 August 2015.

Nursing and Midwifery Council (2011) *The Prepp Handbook* (London: NMC).

Nursing and Midwifery Council (NMC) (2004) *Project 2000 Papers: Counting the Costs – The Final Proposals* (February 1997) (London: Nursing and Midwifery Council).

Odone, C. (2011) 'Sulky, Lazy and Patronising: Finally, We Admit the Existence of the Bad Nurse, the NHS's Dirty Little Secret', *The Telegraph*, http://blogs. telegraph.co.uk/news/cristinaodone/100083415/sulky-lazy-and-patronising-finally-we-admit-the-existence-of-the-bad-nurse-the-nhss-dirty-little-secret/, accessed 4 August 2011.

Ogier, M. E. (1982) *An Ideal Sister? A Study of the Leadership Style and Verbal Interactions of Ward Sisters with Nurse Learners in General Hospitals* (London: RCN).

Orton, S. (2011) 'Re-thinking Attrition in Student Nurses', *Journal of Health and Social Care Improvement*, February: 1–7.

Parliamentary and Health Service Ombudsman (PHSO) (2011) *Care and Compassion? Report of the Health Service Ombudsman on Ten Investigations into NHS Care of Older People* (London: The Stationery Office).

Patients Association (2010) 'Listen to Patients, Speak Up for Change', Patients Association, www.patients-association.org.uk/wp-content/uploads/2014/08/Patient-Stories-2011.pdf, accessed 15 September 2011.

Patterson, C. (2012). 'Reforms in the 1990s Were Supposed to Make Nursing Care Better. Instead There's A Widely Shared Sense That This Was How Today's Compassion Deficit Began. How Did We Come to This?', *The Independent*, 10 April, www.independent.co.uk/voices/commentators/christina-patterson/reforms-inthe-1990s-were-supposed-to-make-nursing-care-better-instead-theres-a-widelyshared-sense-that-this-was-how-todays-compassion-deficit-began-how-did-wecome-to-this-7631273.html, accessed 20 April 2015.

Pembrey, S. E. (1980) *The Ward Sister Key to Nursing: A Study of the Organisation of Individualised Nursing* (London: Royal College of Nursing).

Peters, T. J. and R. Waterman (1982) *In Search of Excellence* (New York: Harvester Wheatsheaf).

Phillips, M. (2011a) 'The Moral Crisis in Nursing: Voices from the Wards', *Daily Mail*, 21 October, http://melaniephillips.com/the-moral-crisis-in-nursing-voices-from-the-wards, accessed 23 February 2012.

Phillips, M. (2011b) 'How Feminism Made So Many Nurses Too Grand to Care', *Daily Mail*, 17 October, http://melaniephillips.com/how-feminism-made-so-many-nurses-too-grand-to-care, accessed 23 February 2012.

Rafferty, A., S. P. Clarke, J. Coles, J. Ball, P. James, M. McKee and L. H. Aiken (2007) 'Outcomes of Variation in Hospital Nurse Staffing in English Hospitals: Cross-sectional Analysis of Survey Data and Discharge Records', *International Journal of Nursing Studies*, 44(2), 175–82.

Royal College of Nursing (2009) *Breaking Down Barriers, Driving up Standards* (London: The Royal College of Nursing).

Salmela, S., K. Eriksson and L. Fagerström (2012) 'Leading Change: A Three-Dimensional Model of Nurse Leaders' Main Tasks and Roles during a Change Process', *Journal of Advanced Nursing*, 68(2): 423–33.

Scott, J. T., R. Mannion, H. Davies and M. Marshall (2003) *Health Care Performance and Organisational Culture* (Oxford: Radcliffe).

Shields, L., P. Morrall, B. Goodman, C. Purcell and R. Watson (2011) 'Care to Be a Nurse? Reflections on a Radio Broadcast and Its Ramifications for Nursing Today', *Nurse Education Today*, 32(5): 614–17.

Smith, P. (2012) *The Emotional Labour of Nursing Revisited*, 2nd edn (Basingstoke: Palgrave).

Studer Group (2006) 'Improve Clinical Outcomes with Hourly Rounding', *Studer Group Newsletter*, 1(7): Sec 1, www.studergroup.com/news, accessed 20 November 2011.

Templeton, S. K. (2004) 'Nurses Are "Too Clever" to Care for You', *The Sunday Times*, 25 April 2004, www.thesundaytimes.co.uk/sto/news/uk_news/article223080.ece, accessed 10 August 2011.

Thomas, J. (2006). *Organisational Culture in Health and Social Care* (London: Radcliffe).

UKCC (1999) *Fitness for Practice: The UK Commission for Nursing and Midwifery Education* (London: United Kingdom Central Council for Nursing Midwifery and Health Visiting).

Ulrich, R., X. Quan, C. Zimring, A. Joseph and R. Choudhary (2004) The Role of the Physical Environment in the Hospital of the 21st Century: A Once-in-a-Lifetime Opportunity, Center for Health Design, www.healthdesign.org/chd/research/role-physical-environmenthospital-21st-century, accessed 10 August 2011.

United Kingdom Central Council for Nursing, Midwifery and Health Visiting (UKCC) (1986) *Project 2000: A New Preparation for Practice* (London: United Kingdom Central Council for Nursing Midwifery and Health Visiting).

United Kingdom Central Council for Nursing, Midwifery and Health Visiting (UKCC) (1985) *Project 2000: Facing the Future* (Project Paper 6) (London: United Kingdom Central Council for Nursing Midwifery and Health Visiting).

van de Glind, I., S. de Roode and A. Goossensen (2007) 'Do Patients in Hospitals Benefit from Single Rooms? A Literature Review', *Health Policy*, 84(2–3): 153–61.

Walshe, K. and J. Higgins (2002) 'The Use and Impact of Inquiries in the NHS', *British Medical Journal*, 325(7369): 895–900.

Walshe, K. and S. M. Shortell (2004) 'When Things Go Wrong: How Health Care Organizations Deal with Major Failures', *Health Affairs*, 23(3): 103–11.

Watson, C. (2012) 'We've All Read about Bad Nurses – Let's Hear It for the Good Ones', The Guardian, 24 September, www.theguardian.com/commentisfree/2012/sep/24/good-nurses-remarkable-people-recognition, accessed 20 August 2015.

West, M. and J. Dawson (2012) *Employee Engagement and NHS Performance* (London: The King's Fund).

West, M. and J. Dawson (2011) *NHS Staff Management and Health Service Quality*. Department of Health, www.dh.gov.uk/prod_consum_dh/groups/dh_digitalassets/documents/digitalasset/dh_129656.pdf, accessed 11 November 2011.

Westmoreland, D. (1993) 'Nurse Managers' Perspectives of Their Work', *Journal of Nursing Administration*, 23(1): 60–4.

Wise, S. (2007) 'Wanted: The Next Generation of Nurse and Midwifery Managers', *International Journal of Public Sector Management*, 20(6): 473–83.

1

Compassion in Care: The Policy Response

Alistair Hewison

Introduction

The failures in care discussed in the introduction and other chapters in this book, while of great concern, are sadly not unique (Martin and Dixon-Woods, 2014). Although the scope and scale of poor quality, particularly at Mid Staffordshire NHS Foundation Trust, were exceptional (Martin and Dixon-Woods, 2014), England is not alone in experiencing organisational crises in healthcare. Similar failures have occured in health systems in New Zealand, the United States and the Netherlands, with several demonstrating the same features as Mid Staffordshire (Dixon-Woods, Baker and Charles, 2013). If the lessons from Mid Staffordshire are to be learned, Martin and Dixon-Woods (2014) suggest that the seemingly straightforward solutions that characterise the problem as arising from poor performance in one hospital, or by 'bad apple' staff be rejected, along with analyses that regard such occurrences as inevitable. The recommended policy response to the events at Mid Staffordshire hospital is set out in three major reports (Francis, 2013; Keogh, 2013; Berwick, 2013) (see below), which discuss in detail the major changes in service delivery that need to take place if compassionate and safe care is to be provided for patients.

The purpose of this chapter is to examine the major recommendations made in these reports and consider them in the context of other developments that have influenced the policy context in which services are delivered and nurses work. This is necessary because to a great extent the shape of nursing is determined by health policy (Hennessy, 2000). However, in the past nurses have had minimal exposure to the study of health policy in their training (Antrobus, Masterson and Bailey, 2004), and it has been suggested that few nurses practising in clinical settings engage in policy debates or perceive health policy to be a 'nursing issue' (Toofany, 2005: 26). Yet nurses work on the 'front line', and their actions can be the crucial factor in whether or not a policy is implemented as intended, because it depends to some degree on the manner in which professionals interpret the policy and incorporate it into their day-to-day work (Barton, 2008: 264). Or to put it another way, from the perspective and experience of the patient, the activity of nurses is, in essence, health policy in action, casting nurses as de facto policymakers at the level of everyday practice (Hannigan and Burnard, 2000). In view of this, it is important to review the current range of policy prescriptions focused on compassion and explore their implications for nursing and healthcare.

The Reports

The year 2013 can be seen as something of a watershed in the history of the English National Health Service (NHS). Three reports were published which delineate the challenge facing the NHS and identify the changes needed if patients' experience and outcomes are to be improved (Woodhead, Lachman and Mountford, 2014). The Francis Report, Keogh Review and Berwick Report were published in February, July and August 2013, respectively, and provide a detailed analysis of the failings at Mid Staffordshire as well as wider quality concerns in the NHS, along with a comprehensive set of recommendations for change and improvement. The Francis Report consists of three volumes and runs to 1782 pages. It makes 290 recommendations (see Figure 1.1 for a summary), and the Inquiry it is based on took three years to complete. The report from the Keogh Review, conducted from 6 February, the publication date of the Francis Report, to July, is 62 pages long and includes eight ambitions (see Figure 1.2). The Berwick Report is 46 pages long and presents ten recommendations (Figure 1.3) focused on the need for improved training and education, and for NHS England to support and spread safety improvement approaches across the NHS. These recommendations were compiled following a study conducted between March and July 2013 of the accounts of contributors to the Mid Staffordshire Inquiry, the recommendations of the Francis Report and others, to distil for Government and the NHS the lessons learned and to specify the changes that were needed. Clearly the material included in these reports is the result of a considerable programme of work; indeed, with a total of 308 recommendations and extensive accompanying commentary it is beyond the scope of this chapter to cover it all. Rather, the approach taken here is as follows:

➤ To summarise the main system problems identified in the reports which in turn had a negative impact on compassionate care.

➤ To focus particularly on the recommendations which identify the need to change the culture from one of targets to one of care.

➤ To identify the challenge for nursing in responding to this raft of policy recommendations.

Why Was There an Absence of Compassion?

The Nursing and Midwifery Council Code of Professional Conduct (2015) requires that registered nurses make the care of people their first concern, treat them as individuals and respect their dignity. However, the factors identified in the reports combined to prevent this being achieved. For example Francis identified the causes of organisational degradation at Mid Staffordshire as systemic; this was manifested in significant weaknesses in NHS systems for oversight, accountability, and a lack of control and leadership (Dixon-Woods et al., 2013). This was primarily caused by a serious failure on the part of the provider Trust Board. It did not listen to its patients and staff or ensure the correction of deficiencies which

---

➤ Foster a common culture shared by all in the service of putting the patient first.

➤ Develop a set of fundamental standards, easily understood and accepted by patients, the public and healthcare staff, the breach of which should not be tolerated.

➤ Provide professionally endorsed and evidence-based means of compliance with these fundamental standards, which can be understood and adopted by the staff who have to provide the service.

➤ Ensure openness, transparency and candour throughout the system about matters of concern.

➤ Ensure that the relentless focus of the healthcare regulator is on policing compliance with these standards.

➤ Make all those who provide care for patients – individuals and organisations – properly accountable for what they do, and to ensure that the public is protected from those not fit to provide such a service.

➤ Provide for a proper degree of accountability for senior managers and leaders, to place all with responsibility for protecting the interests of patients on a level playing field.

➤ Enhance the recruitment, education, training and support of all the key contributors to the provision of healthcare, but in particular those in nursing and leadership positions, to integrate the essential shared values of the common culture into everything they do.

➤ Develop and share ever-improving means of measuring and understanding the performance of individual professionals, teams, units and provider organisations for the patients, the public and all other stakeholders in the system.

Figure 1.1 Summary of the recommendations of the Francis Report.

Ambition 1: We will have made demonstrable progress towards reducing avoidable deaths in our hospitals, rather than debating what mortality statistics can and can't tell us about the quality of care hospitals are providing.

Ambition 2: The boards and leadership of provider and commissioning organisations will be confidently and competently using data and other intelligence for the forensic pursuit of quality improvement. They, along with patients and the public, will have rapid access to accurate, insightful and easy-to-use data about quality at service-line level.

Ambition 3: Patients, carers and members of the public will increasingly feel like they are being treated as vital and equal partners in the design and assessment of their local NHS. They should also be confident that their feedback is being listened to, and see how this is impacting on their own care and the care of others.

Ambition 4: Patients and clinicians will have confidence in the quality assessments made by the Care Quality Commission, not least because they will have been active participants in inspections.

Ambition 5: No hospital, however big, small or remote, will be an island unto itself. Professional, academic and managerial isolation will be a thing of the past.

Ambition 6: Nurse staffing levels and skill mix will appropriately reflect the caseload and the severity of illness of the patients they are caring for and be transparently reported by trust boards.

Ambition 7: Junior doctors in specialist training will not just be seen as the clinical leaders of tomorrow, but clinical leaders of today. The NHS will join the best organisations in the world by harnessing the energy and creativity of its 50,000 young doctors.

Ambition 8: All NHS organisations will understand the positive impact that happy and engaged staff have on patient outcomes, including mortality rates, and will be making this a key part of their quality improvement strategy.

Figure 1.2 Keogh's eight ambitions.

were brought to its attention. It failed to tackle an insidious negative culture characterised by a tolerance of poor standards and a disengagement from managerial and leadership responsibilities. This failure was in part the consequence of too great a focus on reaching national access targets, achieving financial balance and seeking foundation trust status, at the cost of delivering acceptable standards of care (Francis, 2013). So because the managers and leaders of the Trust were striving to achieve a number of targets set by the Government, there was a lack of attention to the fundamentals of care. This was compounded by nursing staff shortages, lack of action when staff raised concerns about care, and a lack of monitoring/

1. The NHS should continually and forever reduce patient harm by embracing wholeheartedly an ethic of learning.

2. All leaders concerned with NHS healthcare – political, regulatory, governance, executive, clinical and advocacy – should place quality of care in general, and patient safety in particular, at the top of their priorities for investment, inquiry, improvement, regular reporting, encouragement and support.

3. Patients and their carers should be present, powerful and involved at all levels of healthcare organisations, from wards to the boards of Trusts.

4. Government, Health Education England and NHS England should assure that sufficient staff are available to meet the NHS's needs now and in the future. Healthcare organisations should ensure that staff are present in appropriate numbers to provide safe care at all times and are well supported.

5. Mastery of quality and patient safety sciences and practices should be part of initial preparation and lifelong education of all healthcare professionals, including managers and executives.

6. The NHS should become a learning organisation. Its leaders should create and support the capability for learning, and therefore change, at scale, within the NHS.

7. Transparency should be complete, timely and unequivocal. All data on quality and safety, whether assembled by Government, organisations or professional societies, should be shared in a timely fashion with all parties who want them, including, in accessible form, with the public.

8. All organisations should seek out the patient and carer voice as an essential asset in monitoring the safety and quality of care.

9. Supervisory and regulatory systems should be simple and clear. They should avoid diffusion of responsibility. They should be respectful of the goodwill and sound intention of the vast majority of staff. All incentives should point in the same direction.

10. We support responsive regulation of organisations, with a hierarchy of responses. Recourse to criminal sanctions should be extremely rare and should function primarily as a deterrent to wilful or reckless neglect or mistreatment.

Figure 1.3 Recommendations of the Berwick Report.

auditing of basic nursing standards and patient care by senior staff to ensure patient needs were met. On one ward, for example, nursing staff appeared to be demotivated and on occasions ignored instructions (with regard to note-taking for example) given by line managers, and there was poor communication between nursing and medical staff (Francis, 2013). There is extensive evidence in the report which charts the further deterioration of standards of nursing in the Accident and Emergency (A&E) Department:

> The culture in the department gradually declined to the point where all of the staff were frightened of the Sisters and afraid to speak out against the poor standard of care the patients were receiving in case they incurred the wrath of the Sisters. Nurses were expected to break the rules as a matter of course in order to meet targets, a prime example of this being the maximum four-hour wait time target for patients in A&E. Rather than 'breach' the target, the length of waiting time would regularly be falsified on notes and computer records. (p. 108)

And one nurse reported:

> I was concerned about the terrible effect that our actions were having on patient care. I did raise this with Sisters [X] and [Y], however their response was extremely aggressive, basically telling me that they were in charge and accusing me and anyone else who agreed with me of not being team players. (p. 108)

In sum, there was an engrained culture of tolerance of poor standards, a focus on finance and targets, denial of concerns, and isolation from practice elsewhere (Francis, 2013). This resulted in compassion not being shown to patients because staff were working in an environment of fear where concerns were ignored, and so were constrained in their efforts to deliver care. In response, it was recognised that the system requires a common positive safety culture, one which aspires to cause no harm to patients and to provide adequate and, where possible, excellent care and a common culture of caring, commitment and compassion (p. 1357).

Following on from the Francis Inquiry, Professor Sir Bruce Keogh, National Medical Director for the NHS in England, was commissioned by the Secretary of State for Health to conduct a review into the quality of care and treatment provided by hospital trusts with persistently high mortality rates. The rationale for this was that high mortality rates at Mid Staffordshire NHS Foundation Trust were associated with failures in all three dimensions of quality – clinical effectiveness, patient experience and safety – as well as failures in professionalism, leadership and governance. Fourteen trusts were selected for investigation based on the fact that they had higher than normal death rates (as measured by the Summary Hospital-Level Mortality Index (SHMI) or the Hospital Standardised Mortality Ratio (HSMR) (Keogh, 2013). It was found that there was a deficit in the high-level skills and sophisticated capabilities necessary at board level to draw insight from the available data and then use them to drive continuous improvement. Too often, boards focused on data that reassured them they were doing a good job, rather than pursuing data that revealed problems, and thereby missed opportunities for improvement. The trusts concerned were isolated and did not have access to the latest clinical, academic and management thinking, and staff did not follow the latest best practice.

With regard to nursing, there were inadequate numbers of staff in a number of ward areas, particularly outside of 'normal' working hours, at night and at the weekend, which was compounded by an over-reliance on unregistered support staff and temporary staff, and this had an impact on care. He also expressed concerns that junior nurses were not valued or supported and argued that 'their energy must be tapped not sapped' (p. 5), found nurses had difficulties accessing senior staff for advice and guidance, and that clinical nursing leadership needed to be strengthened in some of the trusts. Furthermore, staff were not as engaged as they wanted or needed to be (Keogh, 2013), despite the evidence demonstrating that staff who feel valued and engaged provide safer and more compassionate care (Ham, 2014). In addition to the eight ambitions identified, it was concluded that trusts need to be helped to develop cultures of professional and academic ambition, and in particular they need help to establish networks with leading organisations within and outside the NHS to help them to counter the effects of the isolation described above (Keogh, 2013). The themes of leadership and culture are also central to Berwick's analysis of the problems of the English NHS (2013).

The purpose of the Berwick (2013) Report, as noted earlier, was not to analyse in detail what went wrong at Mid Staffordshire, rather, it was to draw out the lessons for the NHS more widely. Indeed, its premise was that it is now time to move on (p. 7). There is also acknowledgement that the NHS is not unsound in its core: its achievements are enormous, and its performance in many dimensions has improved steadily over the past two decades. However, seven main problems were identified by the committee chaired by Berwick, and a set of recommendations (see page 28) developed in response. In summary, the problems were that patient safety was not a central concern throughout the NHS; the tendency to blame staff for system failings, rather than addressing the working arrangements which do not provide them with the conditions for success; the lack of focus on patient care; ignoring warning signals of poor care; diffuse responsibility for care; that the capability to measure and continually improve the quality of patient care needs is not taught or learned; and that fear among staff impedes improvement in complex human systems such as healthcare organisations.

The key messages from the Berwick Report are that the external pressures on the system, such as the need to meet targets, can result in people who work in healthcare organisations losing sight of what should be their primary purpose – namely patient care. Although this may be surprising and disappointing, Berwick's review explains how it can happen. This is also explored in more detail in Chapter 9. Berwick gives particular emphasis to the means of overcoming such failures, concluding that the most important single change in the NHS in response to his report is for it to become, more than ever before, a system devoted to continual learning and improvement of patient care, top to bottom and end to end (Berwick, 2013: 5).

However, this requires a change in culture and leadership. For example leadership involves presence and visibility. Leaders need first-hand knowledge of the reality of the system at the front line, and they need to learn directly from, and remain connected with those for whom they are responsible. Culture change and continual improvement come from what leaders do, through their commitment, encouragement, compassion and modelling of appropriate behaviours (Berwick, 2013: 8). On pages 37–38 of the report, a series of points for action are addressed specifically to the Government, leaders of the NHS, regulators, staff, and patients and their families. This indicates how reports such as those summarised here are designed in part to influence policy. In drawing the attention of policy-makers to the recommendations, the intention is that they will make the changes necessary to ensure compassion is a central feature of care provided by the NHS.

The Government Response

The prominence of compassion as a policy issue is reflected in the document which outlines the Government's initial response to the Francis Report. For example in the foreword, the Secretary of State for Health Jeremy Hunt states, 'I have written to the Chairs of all NHS Trusts asking them to hold events where they listen to the views of their staff about how we safeguard the core values of compassion as the NHS gets ever busier' (DH, 2013b: 6). In this way, direct action to make changes is advocated as part of the policy approach. The response document also acknowledges that the key to providing safe, effective and compassionate care to patients is supporting and valuing staff (p. 31); and that working in health and care is inherently emotionally demanding, and if staff are to be supported to act consistently with openness and compassion, teams need to be given time and space to reflect on the challenging emotional impact of health and care work (p. 31). It also refers to restorative supervision (see Chapter 10) as a best practice example of how to achieve this, and highlights the role of *Compassion in Practice*, the chief nurse's strategy for nursing (DH, 2012), as a key part of its programme for change (see below). The familiar themes of culture change and leadership are evident in the Government's early response. These are developed further in the full report (DH, 2014), which also takes account of the Keogh Review and Berwick Report, summarised earlier, with the secretary of state emphasising that the responses to the Inquiry's recommendations seek to build and strengthen a culture of compassionate care, looking to an NHS future in which world-class leaders working with highly skilled and caring staff consistently strive to improve the care they give to patients (p. 3). In order to do this, 72 actions are presented, organised under the following headings:

> Preventing problems

> Openness and candour

> Listening to patients

> Safe staffing

> Detecting problems quickly

> Taking action promptly

> Ensuring robust accountability

> Ensuring staff are trained and motivated.

These summarise a combination of new measures to support compassion, a range of means of monitoring and inspection to ensure compliance with policy, and a re-statement of fundamental principles and values. For example the Department of Health has commissioned a programme of work from NHS Employers that will provide tools and training for employers to promote the engagement, health and well-being of their staff (p. 15), which in turn should enhance their ability to provide compassionate care. However, from January 2014, the Care Quality Commission will rate hospitals' quality of care in bands ranging from outstanding to inadequate (p. 15), indicating a commitment to inspection and punishment if standards are not met remains. Also the NHS Constitution is seen to take priority, with its central value of putting patients first as the overriding ethos of everything the NHS does (p. 27), to guide policy. The Constitution has compassion as one of its core values; it states: 'We respond with humanity and kindness to each person's pain, distress, anxiety or need. We search for the things we can do, however small, to give comfort and relieve suffering. We find time for those we serve and work alongside. We do not wait to be asked, because we care' (DH, 2010: 12). In this way, the extensive programme of policy action the Government sets out in response to the reports discussed earlier is designed to change practice through application of a range of approaches, some designed to support staff, some to monitor and some to penalise. The policy context nurses must work in is usefully summarised on p. 36 of the report (DH, 2014): 'Systematically creating an environment in which compassionate care is the norm requires imaginative commissioning, organisational commitment, planning, education, training, reinforcement through leadership, and insightful scrutiny and challenge. It is the opposite of the "soft" issue it is too often characterised to be.' Ensuring compassionate care is therefore not just one 'issue' for organisations providing care to address; rather it is, along with safety, the essence of the business that they are in. Another element of this policy framework, referred to in the response, is *Compassion in Practice* (DH, 2012), which is examined here because of its particular relevance for nursing.

Compassion in Practice

Chief Nurse Jane Cummings began work on a strategy for nursing in 2012. She reported that her starting point for this work was to itemise the five areas she believed defined good nursing, which she called 'the five Cs':

> ➤ Care and compassion in how we look after patients
> ➤ Courage to do the right thing, even if it means standing up to senior people to act for the patient's best interests
> ➤ Commitment to our patients and profession
> ➤ Communicating well at all times. (Cummings, 2012)

These were later supplemented with the addition of a further 'C' – competence (DH, 2012) – as part of the Compassion in Practice strategy document produced by the chief nurse. It is noted in the strategy that the values and behaviours covered by the six Cs are not, in themselves, new (DH, 2012: 13), nor is the approach to characterising nursing as being made up of a number of components. Indeed, in the 1980s five and later six Cs were identified by Roach (1984, 1987, 2007). These were compassion, competence, confidence, conscience, commitment and comportment (added later).

The purpose of this policy document is to set out the shared purpose for nurses, midwives and care staff to deliver high-quality, compassionate care and to achieve excellent health and well-being outcomes (DH, 2012: 7). This has been accompanied by a series of events and initiatives (see www.england.nhs.uk/nursingvision/), and progress has been reported in a number of areas based on reports from practitioners (DH, 2013a). However, this strategy has not been universally welcomed. For example the reductionist approach of identifying six elements of a compassionate culture may result in people planning 'quick fixes' for each of the six values and not considering the entire system and context in which care takes place (Dewar and Christley, 2013). Furthermore, Dewar and Christley argue, it is disappointing that the vision and strategy are limited to healthcare staff and exclude the wider team and associated collaborative working (Dewar and Christley, 2013: 48). Similarly, the focus on nursing has been questioned by Cornwell (2012), who found it troubling because of its attempt to create a vision for nursing, midwifery and care giving which seems to be seen as separate from the rest of the healthcare system. She argues that it is not possible to deliver reliable, compassionate care unless it is a central concern and overriding commitment of the whole system (Cornwell, 2012), and based on the findings from a systematic literature review, Flynn and Mercer (2013) conclude that if the NHS is suffering from a compassion deficit, then this is more likely to be due to the political ideology driving current health policy, and not due to any shortcomings in the caring values of nurses (p. 14). The impact of the wider context is also highlighted by Crawford et al. (2011), who observe that in the target-driven pressurised culture of healthcare, where individual practitioners are intensively audited and monitored, and whose jobs hang in the balance, the very thing that healthcare aspires to – caring for people – may be severely compromised. In light of this, it would seem the compassion in practice policy requires further development to articulate a clear vision of the types of compassionate practice healthcare staff should be aiming towards. It does not explicitly state this in the vision and requires healthcare staff to work hard to extract the main messages (Dewar and Christley, 2013).

The other issue that is not completely resolved in the policy documents referred to here is staffing levels. *Compassion in Practice* (DH, 2012) recommends use of national and local evidence to provide tools to determine, locally, the most appropriate staffing levels for a particular health and social care setting that reflects and delivers quality of care, productivity and a good patient or user experience. Francis (2013) called for standard procedures and practice to include evidence-based tools for establishing what each service requires as a minimum in terms of staff numbers and skill mix, including nursing staff on wards, and that this should be monitored by the NHS Litigation Authority. This becomes a considerable challenge when it is considered there is no definitive agreement on safe staffing levels. Similarly, Berwick (2013) advocates that the Government, Health Education England and NHS England should assure sufficient staff are available to meet the NHS's needs now and in the future, and that healthcare organisations should ensure that staff are present in appropriate numbers to provide safe care at all times. This should involve determining staffing levels in accordance with scientific evidence on safe staffing, adjusted to patient acuity and the local context, including nurse-to-patient staffing ratios, and skill mix between registered and unregistered staff (Berwick, 2013). In the Keogh Review (2013), the statistical analysis performed showed a positive correlation between inpatient-to-staff ratio and a high HSMR score (p. 21), and Ambition 6 (see Figure 1.2) again recommends attention be given to staffing levels. Yet local application of staffing tools is irrelevant if there are insufficient nurses, with the right skills, available to be deployed locally (RCN, 2013). Moreover, it has been observed that seven and a half minutes per patient per hour is the amount of time available when the staffing ratio on a ward is one registered nurse to eight patients, and this makes it difficult to deliver safe care (Osborne, 2014). Similarly, Ball et al. (2014) found that nurses reported being unable to comfort or talk with patients and update nursing care plans because they did not have enough time during their shifts. Consequently, the ability of healthcare staff to demonstrate compassion may be as much a function of staffing levels, and the amount of time staff have to devote to patients, as it is the personality and predisposition of the caregiver (Mannion, 2014). The evidence which demonstrates this association between staffing levels and patient outcomes (Griffiths et al., 2014; Ball et al., 2012; Aiken et al., 2002; Rafferty et al., 2007) provides the basis on which the Safe Staffing Alliance (www.safestaffing.org.uk/) is lobbying for statutory minimum staffing levels; it argues these levels must be respected as a minimum, not a ceiling, and if levels fall below the minimum, this should be reported and corrected. The Royal College of Nursing has also addressed this issue, making specific recommendations about care of older people and maintaining, for example, that for basic safe care the overall staffing levels should not drop below one staff member to 3.3 to 3.8 patients (depending on acuity). This means that on a typical 28-bed ward, at least eight staff would be required on duty, with no fewer than four of these being registered nurses (RCN, 2012). Even though trusts are now required to publish their nurse staffing levels (NHS England, 2014) and guidance exists on how to set them (National Institute for Healthcare and Excellence [NICE], 2014), it is a far from straightforward process. Because there is no single nursing staff-to-patient ratio that can be applied across the whole range of wards to safely meet patients' nursing needs, and each ward has to determine its nursing staff requirements to ensure safe patient care (NICE, 2014), the process is complex and involves the analysis of a range of data. So although there is broad acceptance that there is a positive association between higher levels of registered nurses working on wards and patient outcomes there is a lack of agreement on the precise means of determining the 'right' level (Jones et al., 2015). This is likely to remain a hotly debated area of health policy.

In the final part of the chapter, the importance of organisational culture and leadership will be examined. This is necessary because compassion is not just an issue for frontline staff, it should be a concern at all
levels of the organisation from 'bedside to board' (Mannion, 2014: 115),
and staff need support from their organisations if they are to remain
compassionate and reduce patient suffering (Lown, 2014). If the policy
aspiration that compassion becomes central to healthcare discussed earlier
is to be realised, then the evidence suggests fundamental changes will be
required in these two areas in particular.

Organisational Culture and Leadership

This is also recognised in the reports; for example, in addition to safety,
healthcare needs to have a culture of caring, commitment and compassion; however, it cannot be assumed that such a culture is shared by
all who provide healthcare services to patients (Francis, 2013: 1360).
Leadership is about mobilising the attention, resources and practices of
others towards particular goals, values or outcomes. The continual reduction of patient harm requires clarity and constancy of purpose among all
leaders, from the front line to the prime minister, and across the whole
system (Berwick, 2013: 15).

This indicates that if compassionate care is to be provided for
patients, the culture has to be 'right', and good leadership needs to
be demonstrated. However, simply urging people to think differently
is unlikely to overrule the complex forces that shape organisational
behaviour (Davies and Mannion, 2013). Furthermore, although culture
may lie at the root of many health service failings, a more sophisticated
understanding of its dynamics and the role of policy is needed if those
failings are to be addressed (Davies and Mannion, 2013). This presents a
particular challenge because as Konteh et al. (2011) observe, despite its
widespread use and appeal among policymakers, the meaning and definition of organisational culture remains contested (p. 112). Moreover, a
systematic review undertaken by Parmelli et al. (2011) could not identify any effective generalisable strategies for changing organisational
culture.

The policy prescriptions outlined in the reports discussed earlier indicate that major change is required if the culture of the NHS is to become
one focused on compassion. However, there is still some way to go, as
demonstrated in a recent online survey of 2030 staff in the NHS, 33 per
cent of this total being nurses, which found that only 39 per cent felt their
organisation was a place of openness, honesty and challenge (King's Fund,
2014). Forty-three per cent felt swift and effective interventions were not

taken when needed, and 45 per cent felt there was no pride or optimism among staff (King's Fund, 2014). Some of the reasons for this were noted earlier – the lack of staff support and the focus on targets for example – and are explored further in Chapter 9.

If staff are to feel more involved in, and committed to the organisations they work in, then active programmes of staff engagement are required (Ham, 2014), as well as effective leadership. It has been recommended that the type of leadership the NHS requires needs to change, with the old model of 'heroic' leadership by individuals being replaced with shared leadership both within and across organisations (King's Fund, 2011). This is reflected in the extensive leadership development activity taking place in the NHS (Dawson et al., 2009; DH, 2009; NHS Leadership Academy, 2011), which, although welcome, has some limitations with regard to approach and content (Hewison and Morrell, 2014). However, the emphasis on leadership as part of the solution to the compassion deficit in healthcare remains strong (Storey and Holti, 2013; West, 2014).

In setting out what the essential ingredients of the new culture of the NHS should be like, Francis (2013) identified the following:

> ➣ Acceptance that patients' needs come before one's own.

> ➣ Recognition of the need to empathise with patients and other service users.

> ➣ A willingness to provide patients and other service users with the assistance that one would want for oneself, or to refer them to a person with the ability to provide that help.

> ➣ A willingness to listen to patients and service users to discover what they want for themselves.

> ➣ A willingness to work together with others for the benefit of patients and other service users.

> ➣ A commitment to draw concerns about patient safety and welfare to the attention of those who can address those concerns (p. 1360).

If this is to be achieved, then a wide range of approaches will be required, and nurses will be central to this process because, as noted earlier, nurses implement policy in practice. As Berwick observes, only the actions of front-line staff can realise safe compassionate patient care and improvements to the healthcare system (Berwick, 2013: 23), and this will involve action on a number of levels. There is no 'magic bullet' for improving quality in healthcare; rather, improvement requires multiple approaches, including strong leadership, a participatory culture, direction and control, and critical feedback on performance without blame (Dixon-Woods et al., 2014). Getting the right balance of activity in these areas will determine the extent to which nurses are able to deliver compassionate care. The policy context has a direct impact on the environment nurses work in and hence the care they are able to provide.

Conclusion

The definition of quality in healthcare, enshrined in law, includes three key aspects: patient safety, clinical effectiveness and patient experience. A high-quality health service exhibits all three. However, achieving them all ultimately happens when a caring culture, professional commitment and strong leadership are combined to serve patients, which is why the Care Quality Commission is inspecting against these elements of quality (Stevens, 2014: 8). This statement about the direction of the NHS from its chief executive indicates that policy action to address compassion in care takes a number of forms. The reference to the Care Quality Commission by Stevens is significant because it is illustrative of the current pressurised environment of healthcare in which inspection and targets remain a dominant feature in the policy approach. Indeed in a large-scale study of culture change in hospitals, it was concluded that the 'perform or perish' model most closely reflects the current culture of the NHS. It is dominated by a pace agenda and seeks to adopt quick-fix, short-term solutions to what are often long-term and enduring challenges (Patterson et al., 2011). However, if lasting change focused on care is to occur, Patterson et al. (2011) advocate a relational and responsive model that is better suited to address the diverse issues surrounding the provision of high-quality, dignified care which acknowledges the complexities inherent in the delivery of healthcare. If the safety-centred learning culture envisaged by Francis and Berwick is to become a reality, then a major shift in the current policy approach will be required. Until this occurs, nurses will continue to work in an environment that makes it difficult to provide compassionate care. This could perhaps serve as motivation to advocate on patients' behalf, engage with the policy process and bring whatever influence they can to bear shaping future policy in this area.

References

Aiken, L. H., S. P. Clarke, D. M. Sloane, J. Sochaski and J. H. Silber (2002) 'Hospital Nurse Staffing and Patient Mortality, Nurse Burnout, and Job Dissatisfaction', *Journal of the American Medical Association*, 288(16): 1987–93.

Antrobus, S., A. Masterson and J. Bailey (2004) 'Scaling the Political Ladder', *Nursing Management*, 11(97): 23–8.

Ball, J., T. Murrells, A. M. Rafferty, E. Morrow and P. Griffiths (2014) '"Care Left Undone" during Nursing Shifts: Associations with Workload and Perceived Quality of Care', *BMJ Quality & Safety*, 23: 116–25.

Ball, J., G. Pike, P. Griffiths, A. M. Rafferty and T. Murrells (2012) 'RN4CAST Nurse Survey in England', National Nursing Research Unit, www.safestaffing. org.uk/downloads/rn4cast-nurse-survey-in-england, accessed 27 April 2016.

Barton, A. (2008) 'New Labour's Management, Audit and "What Works" Approach to Controlling "Untrustworthy" Professions', *Public Policy and Administration*, 23(3): 263–77.

Berwick, D. (2013) 'A Promise to Learn – A Commitment to Act: Improving the Safety of Patients in England', National Advisory Group on the Safety of Patients in England, www.gov.uk/government/uploads/system/uploads/ attachment_data/file/226703/Berwick_Report.pdf, accessed 30 October 2014.

Cornwell, J. (2012) 'Designing a Culture of Compassionate Care', The King's Fund, 8 October, www.kingsfund.org.uk/blog/2012/10/developing-culture-compassionate-care, accessed 19 November 2014.

Crawford, P., P. Gilbert, G. Gilbert and C. Gale (2011) 'The Language of Compassion', *Taiwan International ESP Journal*, 3(1), 1–16.

Cummings, J. (2012) 'Jane Cummings' Voicepiece: Our Commitment to Improve', 7 August, http://cno.dh.gov.uk/2012/08/07/jane-cummings-voicepiece-3/, accessed 17 August 2012.

Davies, H.T.O. and R. Mannion (2013) 'Will Prescriptions for Cultural Change Improve the NHS?', *British Medical Journal*, 346(1 March): 1–4.

Dawson, S., P. Garside, R. Hudson and C. Bicknell (2009) 'The Design and Establishment of the Leadership Council', NHS Leadership Council, www. dh.gov.uk/prod_consum_dh/groups/dh_digitalassets/documents/digitalasset/ dh_093388.pdf, accessed 1 October 2009.

Dewar, B. and Y. Christle (2013) 'A Critical Analysis of Compassion in Practice', *Nursing Standard*, 28(10): 46–50.

Department of Health (DH) (2009a) *Inspiring Leaders: Leadership for Quality. (Guidance for NHS Talent and Leadership Plans)* (London: DH).

Department of Health (DH) (2009b) 'National Leadership Council: Championing the Transformation of Leadership Across the NHS', www.dh.gov.uk/en/ Aboutus/HowDHworks/BoardsandCommittees/DH_09765, accessed 10 September 2009.

Department of Health (DH) (2010) *The NHS Constitution: The NHS Belongs to Us All* (London: DH).

Department of Health (DH) (2012) *Compassion in Practice: Nursing, Midwifery and Care Staff: Our Vision and Strategy* (London: DH).

Department of Health (DH) (2013a) *Care, Compassion, Competence, Communication, Courage, Commitment: Compassion in Practice – One Year on* (London: DH).

Department of Health (DH) (2013b) *Patients First and Foremost: The Initial Government Response to the Report of The Mid Staffordshire NHS Foundation Trust Public Inquiry* (London: DH).

Department of Health (DH) (2014) *Hard Truths: The Journey to Putting Patients First, Volume One of the Government Response to the Mid Staffordshire NHS Foundation Trust Public Inquiry* (London: DH).

Dixon-Woods, M., S. McNicol and G. Martin (2014) 'Ten Challenges in Improving Quality in Healthcare: Lessons from the Health Foundation's Programme Evaluations and Relevant Literature', *BMJ Quality & Safety*, 21, 876–84.

Dixon-Woods, M., R. Baker, K. Charles, J. Dawson, K. G. Jerzembek, G. Martin, I. McCarthy et al. (2013) 'Culture and Behaviour in the English National Health Service: Overview of Lessons from a Large Multimethod Study', *BMJ Quality & Safety*, 2013(0): 1–10. doi:10.1136/bmjqs-2013-001947.

Flynn, M. and D. Mercer (2013) 'Is Compassion Possible in a Market-led NHS?', *Nursing Times*, 109(7): 12–14.

Francis, R. (2013) *Report of the Mid Staffordshire NHS Foundation Trust Public Inquiry: Executive summary* (London: The Stationery Office).

Ham, C. (2014) *Improving NHS Care by Engaging Staff and Devolving Decision-Making. Report of the Review of Staff Engagement and Empowerment in the NHS* (London: King's Fund).

Hannigan, B. and P. Burnard (2000) 'Nursing, Politics and Policy: A Response to Clifford', *Nurse Education Today*, 20: 519–23.

Hennessy, D. (2000) 'The Emerging Themes', in D. Hennessy and P. Spurgeon (eds) *Health Policy and Nursing Influence, Development and Impact* (Basingstoke: Palgrave Macmillan) 1–38.

Hewison, A. and K. Morrell (2014) 'Leadership Development in the English National Health Service: A Counter Narrative to Inform Policy', *International Journal of Nursing Studies*, 51(4): 677–88.

Jones, A., T. Powell, S. Vougioukalou, M. Lynch and D. Kelly (2015) *Research into Nurse Staffing Levels in Wales* (Cardiff: Welsh Government Social Research), http://orca.cf.ac.uk/73771/1/Nurse%20staffing%20levels%20project%20report%20PUBL%20version.pdf, accessed 21 August 2015.

Keogh, B. (2013) 'Review into the Quality of Care Provided by 14 Hospital Trusts in England: Overview Report', National Health Service, www.nhs.uk/NHSEngland/bruce-keogh-review/Documents/outcomes/keogh-review-final-report.pdf, accessed 30 October 2014.

King's Fund (2014) *Culture and Leadership in the NHS – The King's Fund 2014 Survey* (London: King's Fund).

King's Fund (2011) *The Future of Leadership and Management in the NHS – No More Heroes. Report from The King's Fund Commission on Leadership and Management in the NHS* (London: King's Fund).

Konteh F., R. Mannion and H.T.O. Davies (2011) 'Understanding Culture Management in the English NHS: A Comparison of Professional and Patient Perspectives', *Journal of Evaluation in Clinical Practice*, 17(1): 111–17.

Lee, M. B., L. Tinevez and I. Saeed (2002) 'Linking Research and Practice: Participation of Nurses in Research to Influence Policy', *International Nursing Review*, 49: 20–6.

Lown, B. A. (2014) 'Toward More Compassionate Healthcare Systems', *International Journal of Health Policy and Management*, 2(4): 199–200.

Martin, G. P. and M. Dixon-Woods (2014) 'After Mid Staffordshire: From Acknowledgement, through Learning, to Improvement', *BMJ Quality & Safety*, 23: 706–8.

Mannion, R. (2014) 'Enabling Compassionate Healthcare: Perils, Prospects and Perspectives', *International Journal of Health Policy and Management*, 2(3): 115–17.

NHS England (2014) How to Ensure the Right People, with the Right Skills, Are in the Right Place at the Right Time: A Guide to Nursing, Midwifery and Care Staffing Capacity and Capability, www.england.nhs.uk/wp-content/uploads/2013/11/nqb-how-to-guid.pdf, accessed 20 November 2014.

NHS Leadership Academy (2011) Clinical Leadership Competency Framework, NHS Leadership Academy, www.leadershipacademy.nhs.uk/wp-content/uploads/2012/11/NHSLeadership-Leadership-Framework-Clinical-Leadership-Competency-Framework-CLCF.pdf, accessed 20 September 2014.

National Institute for Healthcare and Excellence (NICE) (2014) Safe Staffing for Nursing in Adult Inpatient Wards in Acute Hospitals, National Institute for Health and Care Excellence, London, www.nice.org.uk/guidance/sg1/chapter/1-Recommendations, accessed 21 August 2015.

Nursing and Midwifery Council (2015) The Code: Professional Standards of Practice and Behaviour for Nurses and Midwives, Nursing and Midwifery Council, London, www.nmc.org.uk/globalassets/sitedocuments/nmc-publications/revised-new-nmc-code.pdf, accessed 20 August 2015.

Parmelli, E., G. Flodgren, F. Beyer, N. Baillie, M. E. Schaafsma and M. P. Eccles (2011) 'The Effectiveness of Strategies to Change Organizational Culture to Improve Healthcare Performance: A Systematic Review', *Implementation Science*, 6(33): 1–8.

Osborne, S. (2014) 'How Can Nurses Show Compassion in 7.5 Minutes an Hour?', Safe Staffing Alliance, www.safestaffing.org.uk/, accessed 20 November 2014.

Patterson, M., M. Nolan, J. Rick, J. Brown, R. Adams and G. Musson (2011) From Metrics to Meaning: Culture Change and Quality of Acute Hospital Care for Older People. Report for the National Institute for Health Research Service Delivery and Organisation Programme, www.nets.nihr.ac.uk/__data/assets/pdf_file/0003/64497/FR-08-1501-93.pdf, accessed 25 November 2014.

Rafferty, A. M., S. P. Clarke, J. Coles, J. Ball, P. James, M. McKee and L. H. Aitken (2007) 'Outcomes of Variation in Hospital Nurse Staffing in English Hospitals: Cross-sectional Analysis of Survey Data and Discharge Records', *International Journal of Nursing Studies*, 44: 175–82.

Roach, S.M.S. (2007) *Caring, The Human Mode of Being. A Blueprint for the Health Professional*, 4th edn (Ottawa: Canadian Health Association).

Roach S.M.S. (1984) *Caring: The Human Mode of Being, Implications for Nursing, a Monograph* (Toronto: University of Toronto, Faculty of Nursing).

Roach S.M.S. (1987) *The Human Act of Caring, A Blueprint for the Health Professions* (Ottawa: Canadian Healthcare Association).

Royal College of Nursing (RCN) (2013) Safe Staffing Levels – A National Imperative. The UK Nursing Labour Market Review 2013. Royal College of Nursing, London.

Royal College of Nursing (RCN) (2012) Safe Staffing for Older People's Wards. Royal College of Nursing, London.

Stevens, S. (2014) 'Five Year Forward View', www.england.nhs.uk/wp-content/uploads/2014/10/5yfv-web.pdf, accessed 30 October 2014.

Storey, J. and R. Holti (2013) 'Towards a New Model of Leadership for the NHS', NHS Leadership Academy, Open Research Online, http://oro.open.ac.uk/37996/1/Towards-a-New-Model-of-Leadership-2013%20online.pdf, accessed 25 November 2014.

Toofany, S. (2005) 'Nurses and Health Policy', *Nursing Management*, 12(3): 26–30.

West, M. (2014) 'The NHS Needs a Leadership Revolution', *The Guardian*, www.theguardian.com/healthcare-network/2014/may/22/nhs-needs-leadership-revolution, accessed 25 November 2014.

Woodhead, T., P. Lachman, J. Mountford et al. (2014) 'From Harm to Hope and Purposeful Action: What Could We Do after Francis?', *BMJ Quality & Safety*, 23: 619–23.

2

Compassion as a Philosophical and Theological Concept

June Jones and Stephen Pattison

Given its prominence in contemporary discussions about publicly provided healthcare, it is perhaps surprising that the concept of compassion lacks detailed study and analysis. It seems to function as a portmanteau concept, like the word *community*, containing many desirable if underdetermined meanings and being confined to very little that is specific. Even its historical origins and usage have received relatively little attention. This chapter seeks to uncover some of the philosophical and theological roots of compassion, a concept that has become familiar in the NHS drive to improve patient care. We begin by considering current understandings of compassion. We then move to explore how compassion was understood by Aristotle, a prominent philosopher who has shaped much of contemporary Western philosophy and ethics, to see that compassion was understood very differently, perhaps more critically, in the ancient world. Thereafter, we consider Judaeo/Christian understandings of compassion, which have informed much of our contemporary language and assumptions but seem to have had relatively little influence on our contemporary lived experience, in terms of serving as a basis for the kind of community and communal solidarity that is necessary for compassion to be really possible.

We focus on the Judaeo/Christian understanding of compassion because it has shaped healthcare development in the UK. As we now live in a multicultural and multi-faith society, there is need to investigate how compassion is understood and practised by many different groups of people. However, this is a less developed area of study and is beyond the scope of this chapter.

Finally, we explore a contemporary ethical framework, the ethics of care, which focuses on the need for compassionate reciprocal relationships. Throughout this chapter, we analyse how the concept of compassion, as variously understood through time, sits uneasily with the call for more compassion within the NHS, as reflected in the Francis Report (Francis, 2013).

The word *compassion* comes from the Latin *compassionem*, meaning 'sympathy' and 'to feel pity'. The word is derived from *com-*, 'together', and *pati-*, 'to suffer'. Thus in its purest form, it denotes the sense of suffering with those who suffer. The use of the word *compassion* is not neutral; it is intrinsically bound up with notions of human relationships and what is expected of them (van der Cingel, 2009). In its contemporary UK English usage, *compassion* can loosely be understood to have some or all of the following meanings and implications in undefined measure:

➤ Sympathy

➤ Pity

➤ Putting oneself in the shoes of another

➤ Feeling with others

➤ Feeling for others

➤ Empathising

➤ Taking others' feelings and situation inside oneself so that their situation impacts upon one's own sense of self and well-being

➤ Solidarity and being alongside another

➤ Suffering with another

➤ Wishing to ameliorate or eliminate others' suffering.

Emotional, imaginative and actively engaged components are each involved in the use of the concept.[1] Consequently, it appears contrary to a cold, distant assessment of the situation of another sentient creature or group of creatures. Rather, it implies a potentially intimate identification with their condition that predisposes to action in coming alongside them and either assisting them to endure or alleviating their situation and suffering.

Although it is most commonly used in the context of individual human relations, compassion can extend from groups to other groups, across species, and indeed across space and time. Thus the charity *Compassion in World Farming* invites active engagement with the present and future plight of thousands of animals transported round the world in the interests of providing cheap food for humans (www.ciwf.org.uk/). At the core of the concept lies some underdetermined but deeply felt kind of intimate, action-guiding and attitude-shaping relational concern that transcends personal boundaries and notions of individualistic isolation based on absolute autonomy to engage warmly, mostly with need and suffering, whether or not the compassionate 'agent' has been invited to help and engage by the 'object' of his or her compassion. The potentially spontaneous, unbidden, even uninvited arousal of compassion in another, joined with its potential for breaching norms and bounds of individual sovereignty and autonomy, might sometimes be gratuitous, invasive and paternalistic. So, for example, a carer might hasten to help someone who appears to be struggling or in difficulty, only to find that the person actually wants to be left alone to sort out his or her own situation or problem. Thus compassion may not always be invited or welcome, despite common assumptions that more of it would be desirable in healthcare.

Is Compassion a Virtue? Challenges and Understandings from the Ancient Philosophical Tradition

In contemporary discussions about the need to deliver more humane healthcare, compassion is often presented as a virtue, a quality found innately or as a product of training within a good nurse (Schantz, 2007; Catlett and Lovan, 2011). Contemporary virtue ethics and the importance of character stem from the ancient philosophical traditions often most closely associated with Aristotle (Nussbaum, 2009). One would expect, then, to see compassion on Aristotle's list of the virtues, qualities to be found in the virtuous person living a good life. However, it is conspicuous by its absence. In *Nicomachean Ethics* (a book dedicated to his son, Nicomachus), Aristotle outlines what virtues people (actually men in his context) need to live a good, flourishing life – a life lived in community with other flourishing beings. He lists qualities such as courage, self-control, patience and truthfulness (*Nicomachean Ethics, Book II, 1106b1–1108b10*). The fully virtuous person takes pleasure in the exercise of these virtues; they bring personal pleasure and serve as ways of bringing pleasure to others. So why didn't he consider compassion necessary as a virtue?

The answer comes in another of his works, *Rhetoric*. The closest we get to compassion is where he discusses pity (*eleos*): what causes it, whom it is felt towards and what state of mind it elicits. Pity is 'a feeling of pain caused by the sight of something evil, destructive or painful, which the person does not deserve to have inflicted on them, and which could happen to us or someone close to us' (*Rhetoric* 2:8). This definition requires that we are motivated in response to what we see others experiencing, something they didn't deserve and something which we would not wish to experience or have inflicted on those we are close to. At least one reason why there is so much public sympathy when a child is abducted is precisely because we know that it could happen to our children or the children of our family and friends.

This definition poses two challenges to contemporary understanding about compassion in healthcare. First, desert is a contentious issue because it requires that we make judgements about which people are more or less deserving of the ill health they are experiencing, and also that we make judgements about who is more or less deserving of the resources necessary to alleviate suffering. Patients are urged to adopt healthy lifestyles by taking more exercise, eating a balanced diet and refraining from substances which are harmful to health. Thus, we may naturally feel more pity for an 8-year-old child with inoperable lung cancer than an 80-year-old adult who has smoked all of her life. Contemporary calls to increase compassion in the NHS take no account of our natural tendency to feel different levels of compassion towards different patients and patient groups, expecting us to overcome what might be seen as 'unprofessional judgements'. Nussbaum notes that we ought to make a distinction between compassion and mercy. Compassion is the appropriate response when faced with undeserved suffering, whereas mercy is the appropriate response when faced with deserved suffering (Nussbaum, 2001). It is not clear whether this distinction is helpful within a health service context. Nurses are probably not stopping to consider whether it is compassion or mercy they are feeling, or meant to be feeling, because the act of caring is more important than analysing the motivation for the care. In palliative care for end-stage liver disease, it matters little whether the care is delivered from compassion towards the person who never took alcohol, or delivered from mercy towards the alcoholic. The most important factor is that good-quality care is provided to both patients.

The second challenge to Aristotle's understanding of compassion comes from his link between pity and the way we feel about those with whom we are in close relationships. The response of pity seems most closely linked to envisaging those closest to us being afflicted with an undesirable state. In healthcare, nurses are being asked to be compassionate towards complete strangers, a form of occupational compassion, rather than familial compassion grounded in deep reciprocal relationships.

There is, however, a more significant reason why compassion is not on Aristotle's list of the virtues. Virtues are qualities that we take pleasure in, and we could never take pleasure in compassion. Compassion is costly because it is painful to experience, and insofar as it is a deep response to the suffering of others, something we seek to avoid because we wish that they were not suffering in the first place. We might value the comfort achieved by effective compassion, but that is not the same as taking pleasure in compassion itself. We value it for its outcome, not its essence. The emotional cost of experiencing occupational compassion can have negative implications on personal, family and institutional life. This would have to be balanced against any desirable outcomes of exercising compassion. If a nurse is compassionate in work to the extent that when he goes home to his family, he has nothing left to give in terms of support to his partner and children, then the cost of being compassionate is too high.

Compassion within Judaeo/Christian Communities

The origins of compassion emerged in social contexts very different from our own, where group identity, solidarity and survival were much more important than individual autonomy or self-determination. The origins of the practice of compassion are communitarian. In communitarian societies, such as those found in contemporary Melansia and in the lands of biblical times, which are composed of 'dividuals' (those who share and rely on each other on a society level) rather than 'individuals', a ready identification with others of the same group, with a concomitant willingness and obligation to help them, would be both necessary and acceptable (Malina, 1983, 1996; Strathern, 1988).2 It was in such societies that Judaism and Christianity emerged, and it is within these traditions that we begin to see compassion described, valued and demonstrated.3

Compassion in the Old Testament is one of a number of important attributes of God that also include justice and mercy (see, e.g., Ps 86.15, Lam 3.22–23). It remains so today in the Abrahamic religions of Judaism, Christianity and Islam. God has mercy or compassion primarily on God's people, but also on the whole human race. Drawing from the notion of the divine as modelled on the ideal parent, God is seen as being alongside God's people in their need and suffering and so as supporting and caring for them. The main Hebrew word for compassion, *rechamim*, is related to the word for womb, and thus implies intimate family relations (Hughes, 2013: 63). It may also imply that compassion ought to be nurturing, promoting growth towards interdependent flourishing, life and security. The compassionate person treats others as members of her family, as God treats God's family/people/tribe. There is, of course, a possible implication of exclusivity and preferential treatment – identifying others as like us and then treating them as we might treat our families and ourselves. This creates the possibility of identifying the 'alien' as not worthy of our compassion.[4]

In the New Testament, Jesus is held to exemplify divine compassion in his teaching and healing work. One of the two Greek words used of Jesus having mercy or compassion, *splagchnizomai*, has the implication of being moved to the guts, being moved with anger, 'raging with compassion' (Mark 1.41; cf. Swinton, 2007).[5] The implication here is that Jesus not only has pity on those who are entrapped by disease and illness, in this instance a leper, but is also angered with the powers of evil that he is engaged in combat with in his ministry (cf. Nineham, 1968: 86). In other words, these powers were not understood as metaphysical invisibilities, but rather they existed within social and material forces that diminish and entrap people (Wink, 1984). The Kingdom of God that Jesus proclaims, inaugurates and exemplifies is an earthly realisation of justice, inclusion and care, including care for outsiders as exemplified in the parable of the Good Samaritan (Pattison, 2013: 85–112; Luke 10.29–37).[6] Compassion in the biblical tradition is not passive sympathy but is integrated with other values attributed to a kingly God such as justice and mercy; it has an active social and political application outworking; the personal, social and political were not separable in biblical times.

The compassion for specific humans and for humanity exemplified by Jesus in his miracles and healings, and ultimately by what was taken to be his sacrifice for human benefit by a criminal death on the cross, is transformed into the love (Greek: *agape*) that St Paul advocates as one of the three Christian virtues in I Cor 13. Faith, hope and love belong together. Paul advocates here and elsewhere the bearing of others' burdens that completes the law of Christ (Gal 5.22, cf. Rom 12.15: 'Rejoice with those who rejoice, weep with those who weep'). *Agape* love is self-giving love of neighbour as oneself, particularly within the Christian community (Rom 13.9–10). It also extends beyond that community and to the undeserving ('Love your enemies and pray for those who persecute you; so you may be children of your Father in heaven, for he causes the sun to rise on the bad as well as the good, and sends down rain to fall on the upright and the wicked alike' [Matt. 5.44–45]). In Aristotle's *Rhetoric*, we saw that pity was something one felt towards someone else, about something which one would not want oneself or others close to oneself to experience in the future. In the New Testament, this takes on a different nature. Here, people have compassion towards others, both friend and foe alike, because they have *already* suffered themselves through recognising their separation from God. Restored to relationship with God through Jesus, they also compassionately care for others. God is seen as 'the Father of compassion and God of all comfort, who comforts us in all our troubles, so that we can comfort those in any trouble with the comfort we ourselves received from God' (2 Corinthians 1:3–4). In this context, compassion becomes *agape* love in action in specific situations. So, for example, Christians in the early church are to treat others as if they were themselves the needy Christ ('Inasmuch you did this [compassionate act of feeding, clothing, visiting in prison] to one of the least of these my brothers, you did it to me' [Matt. 25. 31–46; author translation]) and to put others' needs first. When there is poverty or shortage, a collection is taken up for those affected by it to which all are expected to contribute, sharing their riches willingly as a reflection of God's love and the experience of God's grace (Acts 11.29, Rom. 15.25–8, I Cor 16.1–4, II Cor 8.1–4).

Compassion denotes close identification with, and care for, principally those with whom one belongs, producing the danger of exclusivity and bias towards one's own kind at the expense of strangers or outsiders. This bias is mitigated by the equally important principle and practice of justice that introduces elements of fairness and judgement between people and peoples. This combination of compassionate particularity and inclusive justice can be seen as exemplified in the life, works and teachings of Jesus, in his embodied proclamation of God's rule on earth, which includes strangers and outsiders (e.g. in Mark 7.24–31, Jesus casts out a devil from the daughter of a Syro-Pheonician woman, i.e. the child of someone from a different social group). Here it can be seen that compassion has elements of anger and active protest against suffering and oppression within it that transcend merely being attuned to individual needs and situations. This suggests the notion of compassion can be a more critical and actively change-oriented pursuit. Thus, in our contemporary world, it might be that a carer might be motivated to challenge the structures and practices that permit or foster suffering, rather than simply trying to deal with the sufferings of those who have been negatively affected by, for example, poor levels of staffing that cause neglect of basic nursing needs.[7]

Beyond the New Testament, theological teaching about compassion is limited, even as the challenge to enact compassion in imitation of Christ in the world continues. It would seem in this instance the possible importance of the activity is only equalled by a reciprocal lack of theoretical exploration about its nature as a concept. It really is a case of 'Go thou and do likewise' (Luke 10.37). Although there is an extensive literature on the meanings and implications of love (Lewis, 1960; Nygren, 1969; Outka, 1972), it is not clear that it really extends practical understandings of compassion much beyond that already implicit within the Bible. Nonetheless, Christian thought and practice related to healing and care, the practical application of compassion to those within and outside the Christian community, the deserving and the undeserving, have continued to shape and influence institutions, professions and practices in the West up to the present day; hence the dedication of many hospitals to saints and the presence until recently of 'sisters' among the nursing staff (Swift, 2009).

Although specific theological teaching on compassion may be limited, the spiritual roots of nursing, where compassion for the sick and poor is a pre-eminent motivation for the work, are recorded in various sources. For instance, O'Brien charts the spiritual history of nursing from pre-Christian times, right the way through to post-Reformation, modern-day health-care, where the need for compassion has always been key to the role of the nurse in whatever historical period s/he has cared (O'Brien, 2014). The embodiment of the principle of compassion is described by Henderson in his work on the Renaissance hospitals of Italy, where the largely female nursing staff care for the physical and spiritual state of their patients in a way that demonstrates the value of compassion as a motive for nursing (Henderson, 2006).

> They shelter and tend the sick who come to the hospital as they would Christ Himself. They must receive them with their own hands, care for them, console them and warm, feed and wash them with compassion. They must tend their needs and treat them with all care and charity. (Henderson, 2006: 198)

Catherine of Sienna (1347–80), later to become known as the Patroness of Nursing, worked at La Scala Hospital in Sienna, Italy. She was known as a person of great compassion, gladly taking on the care of some of the most difficult and demanding patients, whom other nurses found diffi-cult to manage (Undset, 2009). Her compassionate character served as a model for other nurses to aim towards in their care of the poor and sick. In Chapter 3, Barbara Schofield provides a detailed description of how compassion has been used in contemporary nursing literature. Prominent nurses have continued to shape the practice of nursing, but more recently, theoretical approaches have provided moral frameworks to describe and proscribe certain behaviours and characteristics. We now turn to examine one such theory, the ethics of care.

The Ethics of Care

Outside of narrow and specific religious understandings and enactments of compassion, the concept has continued to gain importance within a contemporary ethical framework often used in nursing. The 'ethics of care' was developed in the 1970s as something of a feminist response to moral-ity which valued abstract decision-making, where the principles of justice, duties and obligations were emphasised as being the most morally rele-vant means of resolving complex problems involved in balancing commit-ments to work and family. Carol Gilligan (1982) noted that women tend to place less emphasis on abstract ethical reasoning and more emphasis on empathy and compassion as ways of responding to dilemmas. Work began on constructing an ethical theory which could show that compassion and empathy were just as valuable as abstract reasoning. Nel Noddings noted that women were in caring roles from early life and were used to and skilled at face-to-face deliberations. Caring relationships were seen as fundamental to human existence and consciousness, with true caring occurring in reciprocal relationships. The one caring and the one cared for have joint obligations to each other, which are acted out differently according to the relevant context in each situation (Noddings, 1984). For instance, the carer has the obligation to provide appropriate levels of care, but the cared-for has a reciprocal obligation not to place unnecessary burdens on the carer by requiring care beyond that agreed to. The normative claim of the ethics of care is that we ought to maintain relationships by contextualising and promoting the well-being of the caregiver *and* care receiver in a network of social relationships where compassion is foundational.

Within nursing, how is the ethics of care to be expressed? Clearly, a decision is necessary to seek compassionate motivation and responses to deal with the suffering of patients and family members. Van der Cingel claims:

> Compassion gives an answer to suffering by acknowledging it. Acknowledgment of suffering gives us a choice of acting and behaving in such a way that it is evident we want the suffering to end. It is necessary to show acknowledgment in a clear and visible way. This can be verbally or non-verbally, in being present or in taking actions – the precise manner in which compassion is showed is not that important. Not to show acknowledgment means that suffering is being ignored, the loss being of no importance. When the loss is of no importance, the value of what is lost, health for example, is also being denied. (Van der Cingel, 2009: 133)

Here we see the difference in approach that the ethics of care brings. It does not direct us into precise actions. Rather, it seeks to preserve and promote compassionate relationships in whatever way is most appropriate for the context. It directs us to consider our motives as directing our behaviour, not our behaviour per se. In that sense, it has much in common with virtue ethics.

If the ethics of care is to continue as an important framework for nursing, the call for more compassion from nurses towards patients must be equalled by the call for more compassion towards nurses from their clients and employers. It is problematic to reduce the ethics of care to a contractual requirement, lacking any reciprocal arrangements which provide for care and compassion towards the caregiver. By emphasising the feminine nature of compassion and empathy, the ethics of care can also be vulnerable to the charge of perpetuating stereotypes of nursing being a female-type employment, something deeply contentious and harmful to the profession. This does, however, mask a deeper and more interesting question: if the call for increasing compassion is to be taken seriously, how might nursing address how different members of the profession can be supported as they seek to be compassionate? (see also chapter 8)

Discussion

Compassion is currently being used as a catch-all word, a filler for the cracks which have been exposed in the care offered by the NHS as exemplified in the Francis Report. A closer examination of the roots and meanings of compassion has shown that it is far from clear what is being called for. Modern healthcare is provided to diverse patient groups from diverse ethnicities, by staff who are themselves from diverse backgrounds. This is seen as a strength of the NHS, but diversity brings with it the need to avoid a 'one size fits all' approach. Calls for compassion need to acknowledge that the way in which compassion is defined and understood will differ across communities. The different ways compassion is most appropriately expressed may mean that compassion cannot be measured or analysed. In some communities, gender differences prevent compassion being shown by physical touch, for instance. This highlights the need for research to be undertaken to comprehend how compassion is to be understood and appropriately demonstrated among diverse patient and staff groups. Marjorie Ghisoni discusses the components of compassion within a mental health context in Chapter 6.

Aspects of the philosophical and theological traditions described here pose important questions about the nature of compassion which are not addressed by a superficial call for increased compassion within the nursing profession, as per the Francis Report. If one were to take at least some of the origins and articulations of compassion seriously, it would become a concept that was much more radical because it would challenge societal views about care as an occupation rather than an interdependent expression of shared humanity. It would also challenge us to be much more serious about the suffering of others, actively seeking to address the causes of suffering which go beyond the biomedical model. This would include a political and situated quest for justice. Indeed, without some clearly articulated understanding of social, interdependent personhood located within a wider frame of values such as community and justice, compassion can be seen to be a ruined tower that has within it little capacity to motivate or inspire. If it is understood to be the activity and responsibility of solitary individuals, it may have limited power to nurture. Compassion in its fullest sense has to be a two-way street in a society that understands the importance and obligations of the reality of interdependence. It is not just something that powerful professionals can deliver or perform for patients seen as isolated individual consumers. Maybe what is hoped for here is some sense of practical empathic altruism, a willingness and capacity to 'do unto others what you would that they would do unto you' (Matt. 7.12). If this is the case, then the active implementation of some kind of everyday moral awareness test, which might be translated into 'Would I like this to be happening to me or my kind, and if not, what should I change about this situation and my behaviour?' might be both realistic and functional.

We have seen that at heart, compassion involves a feeling or emotion which inspires us to reach out in practical ways to those in need. It thus appears that the current request that the NHS becomes 'more compassionate' seems really to be a requirement that staff make more emotional investment in providing care. What is unclear is how this is to be achieved and how those who are unable or unwilling to make this kind of emotional investment will be managed. The emotion of compassion can be seen as a spectrum. Being at either extreme of this spectrum (being far too compassionate or lacking compassion completely) will be harmful for the member of staff in question, patients and relatives, colleagues and the institution as a whole. Compassion fatigue is also a real phenomenon for staff who over-invest emotionally or who are exposed to patient suffering because of the speciality they work in (Rossi et al., 2012). It is also very difficult to ask staff to increase the level of compassion they both feel and demonstrate when the NHS shows little compassion towards the staff it is trying to motivate. Staff are being urged towards compassion while working in environments which are quick to apportion blame, set increasingly hard to reach targets and are often less than compassionate towards staff who are off sick, for instance. If one is not treated with compassion, it can become increasingly difficult to show it to others (Sanders, Hurwitz and Pattison, 2011). Sawbridge explores this theme further in Chapter 8, and Mastracci in Chapter 11, where the need for resilience in engaging in emotional labour is explored.

If the health service fails to secure genuine compassion from its employees, it may be tempted to settle instead for emotional labour, publicly observable facial and bodily displays that have the appearance of something much deeper, which may not necessarily be present. Hochschild (2012) describes the emotional labour of flight attendants, who are employed for their ability to make work look effortless and pleasurable and to suppress irritation and impatience, which would make airline passengers feel uncared for. This is vital to ensure customer satisfaction and secure regular repeat custom in a competitive market. There is a risk that this will become the default setting within the NHS. Some staff will continue to be motivated by and demonstrate genuine compassion, however that is defined. But pressure could well be brought to bear on all staff to show more compassion in a measurable way. One wonders whether this will result in anything deeper than securing customer satis-faction, rather than eliciting genuine compassion. One could also take the idea of emotional labour as the payment of staff to do that which used to be done by the family. In pre-NHS times, family members would have been the primary providers of food, clean clothing and bedding, and would have provided basic nursing care. We have now moved into a time when the fall-out from the Francis Report could well be that we are paying staff to be more compassionate.

If the call to compassion is seen as an invitation to re-vision healthcare as a communal, corporate activity that exemplifies social solidarity, then it is a bold move to reinvent society and social relations that moves back towards the ideals that brought nationalised healthcare into existence in the 1940s (Woodhead, 2012). If, however, it is merely an inchoate cry for more individual kindness, personal effort and responsibility, mostly on the part of women, in a context of the brutal commercialisation of inti-mate life and care, then it is not only inherently cynical in its injustice and unfairness but also essentially hopeless wishful thinking (Hochschild, 2003). Persons and societies shape each other and virtues like justice, care and compassion belong together. Fundamentally, individualistic proce-dural concepts of the self and of justice, now deeply rooted in contem-porary consumer society, are unlikely to enable compassion and solidarity to flourish in anything other than the most minimal and trivial sense (Campbell, 1987). In addition, we must meet the challenge of exploring what compassion looks like in the many diverse communities in the UK, within different cultural and religious groups. An attempt at compassion can be perceived as offensive if made without cultural sensitivity, and it is possible to view a professional as lacking compassion unless we under-stand what other qualities are being drawn upon. A vision of compassion-ate individuals and communities must therefore also include a vision of justice and structures that enable all persons to flourish in solidarity, one with another.

Notes

1. Empathy suffers from similar problems of scope and definition: 'There are almost as many definitions of empathy as there are researchers in the field … the broad concept of empathy includes a number of key features, such as mimicry, emotional contagion, sympathy and compassion' (Jean Knox [2013] '"Feeling for" and "Feeling with": Developmental and Neuroscientific Perspectives on Intersubjectivity and Empathy', *Journal of Analytical Psychology*, 88(4): 491–509, p. 493).

2. Strathern, Marilyn (1988) *The Gender of the Gift: Problems with Women and Problems with Society in Melanesia* (Berkeley: University of California Press). See also Karl Smith (2012) 'From Dividual and Individual Selves to Porous Subjects', *Australian Journal of Anthropology*, 23(1): 50–64.
3. Here we focus on the Judaeo/Christian roots of compassion because those influenced healthcare in UK society. Many religions have compassion as a foundational concept, which has influenced healthcare development internationally. Islam, Hinduism and Sikhism each have very well-developed ways of understanding the role compassion plays between the divine and the created, lived out in human relationships.
4. Exclusivity and withholding compassion from aliens and strangers is prohibited by God (Ex 22:21; Ex 23:9; Deut 10:9, etc.) and by the NMC Code of Professional Conduct.
5. The Hebrew Scriptures, or 'Old Testament', are written in Hebrew and a small amount of Aramaic. Jesus probably spoke Aramaic, but the text of the New Testament is written in the common Greek of the ancient Mediterranean world, with a few Aramaic words remaining in the text.
6. The Parable of the Good Samaritan is often taken in the contemporary Western world as a paradigm of enacted compassion and extenuating care for strangers. In it, a man is assailed, robbed and injured by robbers but then rescued and cared for by a stranger from a completely different religious group after members of his own religion have failed to meet his needs because this would entail impurity. Parables are complex and multifaceted, so they are not straightforward moral exemplars or normative tales. However, this particular parable has been received in the contemporary world very much in this way.
7. See, e.g., S. Pattison (1994) *Pastoral Care and Liberation Theology* (Cambridge: Cambridge University Press).

References

Aristotle (1989) *Rhetoric* (Cambridge, MA: Loeb Classic Library).

Aristotle (2004) *Nicomachean Ethics, Book II, 1106b1–1108b10* (London: Penguin Classics).

Campbell, C. (1987) *The Romantic Ethic and the Spirit of Capitalism* (Oxford: Blackwell).

Catlett and Lovan (2011) 'Being a Good Nurse and Doing the Right Thing: A Replication Study', *Nursing Ethics*, 18(1): 54–63.

Francis, R. (2013) Report of the Mid Staffordshire NHS Trust Public Inquiry, www.gov.uk/government/publications/report-of-the-mid-staffordshire-nhs-foundation-trust-public-inquiry, accessed 28 May 2014.

Gilligan, C. (1982) *In a Different Voice* (Cambridge, MA: Harvard University Press).

Henderson, J. (2006) *The Renaissance Hospital: Healing the Body and Healing the Soul* (New Haven, CT: Yale University Press).

Hochschild, A. R. (2003) *The Commercialisation of Intimate Life* (Berkeley: California University Press).

Hochschild, A. R. (2012) *The Managed Heart: Commercialization of Human Feeling* (Berkeley: University of California Press).

Hughes, T. O. (2013) *The Compassion Quest* (London: SPCK).

Lewis, C. S. (1960) *The Four Loves* (New York: Harcourt Brace).

Malina, B. (1983) *The New Testament World: Insights from Cultural Anthropology* (London: SCM Press).

Malina, B. (1996) *The Social World of Jesus and the Gospels* (London: Routledge).

Nineham, D. E. (1968) *The Gospel of St Mark* (London: A and C Black).

Noddings, N. (1984) *Caring: A Feminine Approach to Ethics and Moral Education* (Berkeley: University of California Press).

Nussbaum M. (1996) 'Compassion, the Basic Social Emotion', *Social Philosophy and Policy*, 13(1): 27–58.

Nussbaum, M. (2001) *Upheavals of Thought. The Intelligence of Emotions* (Cambridge: Cambridge University Press).

Nussbaum, M. (2009) *The Therapy of Desire: Theory and Practice in Hellenistic Ethics* (Princeton, NJ: Princeton University Press).

Nygren, A. (1969) *Agape and Eros* (New York: Harper and Row).

O'Brien, M. E. (2014) *Spirituality in Nursing*, 5th edn (Burlington, MA: Jones & Bartlett Learning).

Outka, G. (1972) *Agape: An Ethical Analysis* (New Haven, CT: Yale University Press).

Pattison, S. (2013) *Saving Face: Enfacement, Shame, Theology* (Farnham: Ashgate).

Rossi, A. et al. (2012) 'Burnout, Compassion Fatigue, and Compassion Satisfaction among Staff in Community-based Mental Health Services', *Psychiatry Research*, 200(2–3): 933–8.

Sanders, K., B. Hurwitz and S. Pattison (2011) 'Tracking Shame and Humiliation in Accident and Emergency', *Nursing Philosophy*, 12, 83–93.

Schantz, M. L. (2007) 'Compassion: A Concept Analysis', *Nursing Forum*, 42(2): 48–55.

Strathern, M. (1988) *The Gender of the Gift: Problems with Women and Problems with Society in Melanesia* (Oakland: University of California Press).

Swift, C. (2009) *Hospital Chaplaincy in the Twenty-first Century: The Crisis of Spiritual Care on the NHS* (Farnham: Ashgate).

Swinton, J. (2007) *Raging with Compassion: Pastoral Responses to the Problem of Evil* (Grand Rapids, MI: Eerdmans).

Undset, S. (2009) *Catherine of Sienna* (San Francisco, CA: Ignatius Press).

van der Cingle, M. (2009) 'Compassion and Professional Care: Exploring the Domain', *Nursing Philosophy*, 10, 124–36.

Wink, W. (1984) *Naming the Powers* (Minneapolis, MN: Fortress Press).

Woodhead, L. and R. Catto (eds) (2012) *Religion and Change in Modern Britain* (Abingdon: Routledge).

Woodhead, L. (2012) 'Introduction', in L. Woodhead and R. Catto (eds) *Religion and Change in Modern Britain* (Abingdon: Routledge), 1–33.

3

Compassion in Nursing: A Concept Analysis

Barbara Schofield

Introduction

In Chapter 2, Jones and Pattison suggest that compassion has become a familiar concept in regard to driving improvements in patient care in the NHS. It is not surprising that in recent years there has been increasing interest in the subject of compassion in nursing. Numerous patient stories featured in public reports and presented by the media illustrate examples of poor care (Alzheimer's Society, 2009; The Patients Association, 2009, 2010, 2011, 2012; Parliamentary and Health Service Ombudsman, 2011), and following the publication of the Francis Report in 2013 (Francis, 2013), scrutiny of the care provided by registered nurses has increased further. Government reports and directives highlight that the care of patients in some hospital and other care settings is less than adequate (Department of Health [DH], 2008, 2009, 2009a, 2012; National Health Service [NHS] Confederation, Age UK and Local Government Association, 2012; Francis, 2013). A common theme in describing this problem is that poor care appears to be associated with a lack of compassion.

In this chapter, I present a concept analysis of compassion in nursing. I chose to apply the Walker and Avant theoretical framework (2011) to guide a PhD research study[1] which aimed to conceptualise the meaning and significance of compassion when delivering nursing care to older people in hospital. The methodology for the study was grounded theory (Corbin and Strauss, 2008), and although some may argue that concept analysis does not lend itself to the grounded theory approach, in my experience it has been an extremely useful framework to guide the process of analysing emerging data. Thus far I have interviewed patients, their families and carers to explore their views of what constitutes compassionate care. The themes that have emerged have provided a point of reference for observations of registered nurses caring for older people on two hospital wards.

In the following sections, I present a concept analysis of compassion in nursing developed by applying the Walker and Avant (2011) model. The model presents a structured, step-by-step approach and has eight stages: (i) selecting a concept; (ii) determining the purpose of the analysis; (iii) describing all uses of the concept; (iv) identifying the defining attributes; (v) discussion of cases (for the purpose of this chapter, I only discuss one case, taken from my research, describing an interview with a former patient); (vi) identifying antecedents; (vii) identifying consequences; and (viii) defining empirical referents (Walker and Avant, 2011). On the face of it, compassion is a simple term; however, a concept analysis provides a mechanism for examining its component parts and demonstrating its inherent complexity. This is necessary because if compassion is to be achieved in practice, we need to have a better understanding of what it is.

Selecting a Concept

Compassion is viewed as an essential component of nursing care, and in recent years the requirement of the nursing profession to deliver compassionate care has been repeatedly re-stated (NHS Confederation, 2008; DH, 2008, 2009, 2009a, 2012; Firth-Cozens, and Cornwell, 2009; The Patient Association; 2009, 2010, 2011, 2012; RCN, 2010; Parliamentary and Health Service Ombudsman, 2011; NHS Confederation, Age UK and Local Government Association, 2012; Francis, 2013). In December 2012, 'The Nursing, Midwifery and Care Staff Vision and Strategy, Compassion in Practice' was launched (Cummings and Bennett, 2012). Although the characteristics of compassionate care within the Compassion in Practice Strategy reflect current theoretical thinking (Maben, Cornwell and Sweeney, 2010; Ballatt, and Campling, 2011; Dewar, 2011), the definition of what is meant by compassion in regard to nursing care remains contentious. Also, as previously suggested by Jones and Pattison in Chapter 2, how compassion can be recognised and measured is still unclear. With this in mind, the concept of compassion in nursing was selected for analysis.

Purpose of Analysis

Walker and Avant (2011) suggest that the purpose of a concept analysis can be determined by asking the question 'Why am I doing this analysis?' The purpose of this concept analysis is to contribute towards developing an understanding of what compassion is in relation to the provision of nursing care for older people in hospital and to explore how it may be recognised in everyday practice.

Much discussion has occurred regarding the significance of compassion in the delivery of nursing care in the media and in policy documents and reports (see Chapter 1, for example). In light of this, it would have been naïve, and indeed impossible, to start my research with no awareness of the concept of compassion, and in particular without an understanding of what compassion in nursing, and the lack of it, look like. An additional aim for undertaking the concept analysis, therefore, was to provide an overview of compassion in nursing as a baseline for my research.

All Uses of the Concept

Walker and Avant (2011) encourage a review of literature and gathering of data from a range of sources, for example from speaking with colleagues. In order to determine all uses of the concept, I approached this in two ways. First, a review of the literature was conducted by searching the following databases: Summon, BNI, CINAHL, PsychINFO, Medline and HMIC. Policy documents and reports were also identified through a variety of websites. Second, I chose to enrich the concept analysis with the emergent data from my research interviews.

Definitions

The Cambridge Dictionary describes compassion as 'a strong feeling of sympathy and sadness for the suffering or bad luck of others and a wish to help them' (Cambridge English Dictionary Online, 2014). The desire to act upon the suffering of others also features in the Buddhist definition of compassion (Michie, 2012), which describes related qualities including kindness, love, patience and generosity. With regard to nursing care, Chambers and Ryder (2009: 2) describe compassion as 'the essence of caring', 'acting in a way that you would like others to act towards you' and 'a profound feeling resulting from witnessing the pain or distress of others'. Gilbert (2010: xiii) defines compassion as 'basic kindness, with a deep awareness of the suffering of oneself and of other living things, coupled with the wish and effort to relieve it'. However, a concept analysis moves beyond brief definition to address the complexity that is inherent in many concepts.

Compassionate Nursing

The debate about what constitutes compassionate nursing is characterised by four main strands. First is the abundance of words used in association with compassionate nursing care, including *kindness, empathy, understanding, caring, person-centred, relationships, knowing the person, being non-judgemental, listening, responding, responsibility, competence* and *advocacy* for example (Burnard, 1997; Deitze and Orb, 2000; Schantz, 2007; Chambers and Ryder, 2009; Cingel, 2009; Gilbert, 2010; Dewar, 2011). In addition, the term *compassion* has been used interchangeably with other concepts such as *caring, sympathy* and *empathy* (Dietze and Orb, 2000; Schantz, 2007; Straughair, 2012). Third is the recognition of suffering and vulnerability with action. Finally, the caring practices described within nursing ethics illustrate values similar to those reflected in compassion theory (Benner and Wrubel, 1989; Burnard, 1997; Benner et al., 2009; Chambers and Ryder, 2009; Cingel, 2009). With this in mind, ethical and professional responsibilities cannot be excluded from the characteristics which underpin compassionate care.

Compassion has been widely discussed in terms of its application in nursing (Dietze and Orb, 2000; Hem and Heggen, 2004; Schantz, 2007; Firth-Cozens and Cornwell, 2009; Chambers and Ryder, 2009; Maben et al., 2010; Dewar, 2011) and has been described as an essential component of nursing care (Dietze and Orb, 2000; Hem and Heggen, 2004; Chambers and Ryder, 2009). In her concept analysis of compassion in nursing, Schantz (2007) suggests that what distinguishes compassion from related qualities such as empathy, sympathy and caring is the intention to act upon the suffering of others. Others support this notion, suggesting that although compassion relates to the human characteristic of emotion, for example demonstrating sympathy or empathy, there is a deliberate dimension which influences the way in which care is delivered (Dietze and Orb, 2000; Firth-Cozens and Cornwell, 2009; Chambers and Ryder, 2009; Maben et al., 2010). Benner (1984) presents evidence of this, describing it as the healing power of compassion. Von Dietze and Orb (2000) propose that this aspect of compassion adds a moral value to caring.

Models of Compassion

The Compassion in Practice Strategy (Cummings and Bennett, 2012) includes compassion as one of six Cs, all of which carry equal weight and contribute to compassionate care. Alongside the values of Care, Competence, Communication, Courage and Commitment, the six Cs are underpinned by Collaboration, to provide a vision for nurses, midwives and care staff in England. The Leadership in Compassionate Care Programme at Napier University in Edinburgh aims to establish compassionate care as an integral aspect of nursing (Dewar, 2011). Key themes emerging from research associated with the programme are as follows:

'Knowing who I am and what matters to me', 'work with me to shape the way things are done' and 'engage in appreciative caring conversations' (Dewar, 2011). Dewar offers seven Cs of appreciative caring conversations: be Courageous; Connect emotionally; be Curious; be Collaborative; Consider others' perspectives; Compromise; and be Celebratory. Courage is described as 'having confidence to act in a certain way and being able to stick up for the principles of personhood' (Dewar, 2011). The notion that courage is essential to delivering compassion is supported by Gilbert (2010). However, his description of courage focuses on one's ability to deal with emotions and situations (Gilbert, 2010: 413–17). He adds that feeling compassion is conducive to our own health and well-being, although it can involve sadness and grief and can be tricky for some people.

Conditions to Support Compassion

The conditions of self-compassion and compassionate organisations are increasingly acknowledged as essential factors influencing the delivery of compassionate care (Gilbert, 2009; Chambers and Ryder, 2009; Ballatt and Campling, 2011; Youngson, 2012). Crawford et al. (2013) examined mental health practitioner perspectives on compassion in healthcare. In particular, they studied the language of compassion. They identified a concept called 'threat stress', a condition experienced by staff when organisations are focused on driving efficiency and targets, often at the expense of compassion. They found little evidence of the use of compassion language. The focus was on paperwork, time and production, indicating an institutional mentality and emotional distancing. They claim that to deliver compassionate care, practitioners require a compassionate mentality and suggest that organisations should pay particular attention to the social context of care delivery.

Compassion as an Inherent Quality

Compassion as an intrinsic personal quality remains a subject of discussion (Schantz, 2007; Johnson, Haigh and Yates-Bolton, 2007; Gilbert, 2010; Ballatt and Campling, 2011), as does the view that compassion can be learned (Burnard, 1997; Schantz, 2007; Chambers and Ryder, 2009; Gilbert, 2010; Youngson, 2012). The identification of compassion as an inherent personal quality is discussed by Schantz (2007), who claims this does not necessarily mean it cannot be role-modelled and learned in the way that many other beliefs and values are. She refers to the belief of the Dalai Lama that everyone has the potential to feel compassion, and suggests that it is an individual's personal choice whether it is applied. Chochinov (2007) claims that healthcare providers arrive at compassion through various channels; for some, this may be a natural disposition or an intuition, while for others it may slowly emerge through experience. These views provoke the question 'Can compassion be learned?' In his book *The Compassionate Mind*, Gilbert (2010) presents a case for the influence of societal change on our ability to demonstrate compassion. He claims that as we move away from the welfare culture of the last century towards a more competitive and business-orientated society, compassion may be seen as weakness (see also Chapter 9). Gilbert relates this to healthcare and acknowledges that those working in healthcare settings may need to relearn the skill of compassion. Although personal values and choice are important factors influencing compassionate care, it could be said that registered nurses have a professional and contractual obligation to provide such care.

Compassion as a Professional Standard

The Nursing and Midwifery Council (NMC) code of conduct (NMC, 2008) states that nurses must treat people as individuals, respect their dignity, treat them kindly and considerately, and act as their advocate. Although the word *compassion* does not feature in the NMC Code, these regulatory standards imply that compassion is a professional requirement for registered nurses in the United Kingdom, and when next revised it is likely the word compassion will be included.[2] More explicitly, the NMC standards for pre-registration nursing education specify the knowledge, skills and learning outcomes with regard to compassion to be included in the education curriculum (NMC, 2010). Thus compassion is viewed as essential in this context. The word *compassion* was included in the Norwegian code of ethics for nurses in 2001. Hem and Heggen (2004) claim that the vulnerability and dependency of patients imposes a moral obligation on nurses to take care of them. In their study of compassion, they conclude that acknowledging compassion in the ethical guidelines for nursing is necessary, but are keen to emphasise that the practice of compassion is demanding, difficult and dependent on individual nurses and the settings they work in. Having summarised all the uses of the concept, as suggested by Walker and Avant, the next stage is to determine the defining attributes. As demonstrated, the concept of compassion in nursing is complex, and the context within which it is described varies widely. If it is to be understood, more clarity is needed regarding the meaning and significance of the concept.

Defining Attributes

The defining attributes are described by Walker and Avant (2011) as those characteristics that are accepted as being essential to the concept. Characteristics frequently associated with the concept of compassion include kindness, empathy, dignity, caring, communication, healing, sympathy and being non-judgemental and person-centred (Burnard, 1997; Dietz and Orb, 2000; Schantz, 2007; Hem and Heggen, 2004; Cingel, 2009; Dewar, 2011; Chambers and Ryder, 2009; Firth-Cozens and Cornwell, 2009; Maben et al., 2010; Dewar and Mackay, 2010; Smith et al., 2010; Gilbert, 2010; Tadd et al., 2011; Youngson, 2012). Qualities including respect, advocacy, commitment and competence are included in professional and ethical descriptions of nursing (NMC, 2008; Cummings and Bennett, 2012). Here I want to focus on the specific concepts that have emerged through the literature review and have been validated in my research interviews.

The concepts of kindness, empathy, dignity and caring feature in numerous theoretical descriptions of compassion (Burnard, 1997; Dietze and Orb, 2000; Hem and Heggen, 2004; Schantz, 2007; Cingel, 2009; Chambers and Ryder, 2009; Firth-Cozens and Cornwell, 2009; Maben et al., 2010; Dewar and Mackay, 2010; Smith et al., 2010; Gilbert, 2010; Tadd et al., 2011; Youngson, 2012). These themes have also emerged through the early stages of my research. Furthermore, the obligation of nurses to uphold moral, ethical and professional standards is seen as an essential ingredient in delivering good care, and many of the characteristics and qualities described in this context reflect those portrayed when discussing compassionate care (Benner and Wrubel, 1989; Burnard, 1997; Benner et al., 2009; Banks and Gallagher, 2009). Finally, for compassion to be present the recognition of suffering, vulnerability or need with an intention to act upon it must be demonstrated.

Kindness

Throughout my research interviews, the word most commonly used to describe compassion was *kindness* (see Chapter 5). *Kindness* is defined in the Cambridge dictionary as 'being helpful and generous, and considering the feelings of others'. Kindness can be viewed as a natural disposition (Clegg and Rowland, 2010). It originates from the words *kin* and *kindred*, implying that it applies within families, groups and communities. Forrest (2011) describes kindness as paying attention to another person while acknowledging his or her situation and point of view. She claims that being kind is to be open and generous, non-judgemental and respectful of the dignity of the other person. It requires that we do not focus on our own needs, but that we concentrate on the needs of others. Forrest suggests that this may lead us to be vulnerable ourselves.

An interesting discussion regarding kindness is presented by Clegg and Rowland (2010), who distinguish kindness from the acts that are expected of professionals such as 'due care'. Although Clegg and Rowland are discussing kindness in the context of education, the principle is transferrable to nursing and healthcare, and indeed to the debate regarding other virtues including compassion. Sayer (2005) claims that virtue concepts such as kindness should be taken seriously because they matter to people as these concepts affect their well-being, which Sayer describes as 'lay normativity'. Clegg and Rowland (2010) propose that it would be useful to capture the views of teachers through the normative lens of kindness to investigate whether and how they can bring kindness to their interactions with students, and to explore the extent to which these are being re-engineered as due care and professional competencies. This could be applied to nursing as it is equally difficult to distinguish what constitutes genuine kindness rather than a duty of care or professional standard.

Empathy

The word *empathy* is often used interchangeably with *sympathy* (Wiseman, 1996). However, Miller and Keane (1989) draw a clear distinction between the two, describing empathy as 'intellectual and emotional awareness and understanding of another person's thoughts, feelings and behaviour, even those that are distressing and disturbing, and sympathy as the sharing of another's feelings and experiences'.

Dinkins (2011) describes empathy as one of the basic building blocks for ethical conduct towards others, adding that without empathy it is difficult for us to understand the needs of the patient, and without it other virtues such as sympathy or kindness would be difficult to apply. She suggests that empathy should be viewed as a practice rather than a feeling or instinct. The RCN (RCN, 2014) pairs empathy with compassion in its collection of the key concepts that constitute person-centred care. The notion of understanding the needs of the person is similar to descriptions of compassion.

Dignity

Human dignity has been described by Milton (2013) as the 'noble presence of worth'. He claims that in acknowledging the suffering of another, dignity is strengthened. The RCN (2008) states:

Dignity is concerned with how people feel, think and behave in relation to the worth or value of themselves and others. To treat someone with dignity is to treat them as being of worth, in a way that is respectful of them as valued individuals ... when dignity is present people feel in control, valued, confident, comfortable and able to make decisions for themselves. When dignity is absent people feel devalued, lacking control and comfort ... (no page number)

Dignity is closely aligned to compassion. For example in his ABCD of dignity conserving care, Chochinov (2007) presents compassion as one of four core components of dignity alongside attitudes, behaviours and dialogue. Compassionate care is a key feature in both the RCN dignity campaign (RCN, 2009), and the more recent dignity report for consultation (NHS Confederation, Age UK and Local Government Association, 2012).

Ethical, Moral and Professional Obligations in Delivering Compassionate Care

To add another dimension to this complex component of nursing, the ethics of caring is widely acknowledged as being key to the delivery of compassionate care (Benner and Wrubel, 1989; Burnard, 1997; Benner et al., 2009; Chambers and Ryder, 2009; Cingel, 2009). Benner et al. (2009) suggest that ethical obligation, taking into consideration the person's rights, and promoting autonomy and beneficence are what constitute an expert nurse. They claim that the ethic of care must be learned experientially and describe this as ethical comportment: 'the embodied skilled know-how of relating to others in ways that are respectful, responsive and supportive of their concerns'. They add that comportment refers to more than just words, to include intents, beliefs, values, thoughts and feelings that are fused with physical presence and action (Benner et al., 2009: 280). To become an expert nurse, one should feel concern, not indifference; to acquire ethical expertise one must have the talent to respond to those ethical situations to which ethical experts would respond, and one must have the sensibility to experience satisfaction or regret at the outcome of one's action. The authors claim that in a field where caring practices are central (including protection of the vulnerable), it is difficult, if not impossible, to have encounters that do not encompass both clinical and ethical expertise.

The defining attributes of compassion in nursing identified in this concept analysis include kindness, empathy, caring, dignity, upholding professional conduct and practice in order to protect people from harm, consider their rights and promote autonomy and beneficence; and recognition of a need for care, with a wish to do something about it (see Figure 3.1). In the next

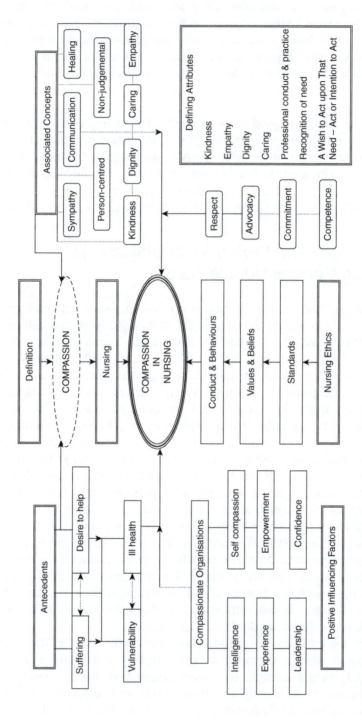

Figure 3.1 Concept map: Compassion in nursing.

section, a case study drawn from my research is used to demonstrate how these defining elements of compassion are identified by patients and carers.

The Cases

Walker and Avant (2011) recommend using model, borderline, related, contrary, invented and illegitimate cases. Although I have analysed all the recommended cases, for the purpose of this chapter I only include the model case, which presents the reflections of an elderly gentleman who had previously been a patient in hospital. He was invited to talk about compassionate nursing care. He and a patient he describes have been anonymised by the use of pseudonyms.

Model Case

According to Walker and Avant (2011), a model case is an example that features all of the defining attributes:

Jim had been a patient on an acute surgical ward. In this reflection, he is describing the care provided by a registered nurse to an elderly gentleman called Stanley. They were situated in a four-bedded bay along with two other gentlemen. Jim acknowledged that Stanley had become very confused on the ward, and he and his fellow room occupants had been quite impatient with, and about, him. When referring to Stanley's behaviour with the nurses who were caring for him, Jim said, 'He was quite rude to them, aggressive even.'

Jim reflected on the events of previous days, and in particular how one of the nurses had involved himself and the other patients in loudly trying to 'jolly' Stanley along. He explained that on one particular day, another nurse who was looking after Stanley had spoken with kindness in her voice. He overheard her explaining to Stanley that she was there to help him:

> The nurse was obviously looking after him properly. He was using this foul language, but I think she can understand the man needs help, he is suffering and he is confused. That must be a form of compassion and she didn't discuss it with any one of us patients.

Having previously heard the nurses shouting out at Stanley, the approach from this nurse impressed Jim as he realised that she was understanding of his situation and was diplomatic in her response to him. He reflected how previous encounters had influenced his own negative attitude towards Stanley, and that of his fellow patients. It appeared that although this nurse had not discussed Stanley with them, the professional, caring and empathetic approach of the nurse had led them to empathise with Stanley also.

Jim then described how the following day the nurse had offered to look after Stanley, even though she was not delegated to do this. Jim perceived that the nurse had offered to do this because she was stronger than the nurse who should have been looking after Stanley:

> Then next day, she was bigger than the other nurse (this nurse had been assigned to look after Stanley) and she said 'I'll do Stanley.' To me, she was brilliant.

When asked if the nurse had needed to be bigger and stronger, Jim denied any observation of physical intervention. He explained how the nurse had calmed Stanley. In reality it is more likely that she recognised the importance of continuity and knew that she could offer some degree of familiarity for Stanley. She had understood his situation and had no hesitation in offering to care for him again. In doing this, she had demonstrated empathy, kindness and caring. The most significant feature of this story is the silent impact this nurse had on how the other patients perceived and reacted to Stanley. Jim told me that as a direct result of her approach to Stanley, he and his fellow patients became helpful and understanding towards Stanley. From this perspective, the nurse had protected Stanley's dignity; her discretion had upheld professional conduct; her practice had respected the rights to confidentiality and privacy, and in doing so she had safeguarded him from harm and promoted his autonomy and beneficence. He was now socially accepted in his environment, and his recovery was remarkable.

Antecedents

The widely recognised condition required in order that compassion can take place is suffering, or the threat of suffering (Schantz, 2007; Gilbert, 2009; Chambers and Ryder, 2009; Michie, 2012). In the context of healthcare and nursing, this is expanded to include illness or risk of illness, and human vulnerability (Hem and Heggen, 2004; Cingel, 2009; Gilbert, 2009; Dewar, 2011; Youngson, 2012). Although I acknowledge that illness, suffering and vulnerability are conditions required to prompt compassionate nursing, it would be short-sighted not to consider other factors which may enable compassion. Understanding and reflecting on the nature of compassion has led me to consider two aspects of compassion theory as antecedents for compassionate nursing: these are self-compassion and compassionate workplace culture.

Suffering

Suffering has been described as 'an experience characterised by a loss of control that creates insecurity and a feeling of being trapped in the circumstances of suffering' (Ferrell and Coyle, 2008: 108). Milton (2013) suggests that human suffering is an individualised, subjective and complex lived experience that potentially presents in situations as ethical dilemmas.

In her concept analysis of self-compassion, Reyes (2012) suggests that suffering manifests as a pattern of decreased self-care, decreased ability to relate to others and diminished autonomy. She describes six realms of suffering as 'states of being' experienced as an event, a situation, an emotional reaction, a psychological condition, spiritual alienation or a physical response to illness or pain.

Vulnerability

The alleviation of vulnerability is essential to delivering good care (Benner et al., 2009; Banks and Gallagher, 2009). A commonly cited reason for the need for professional ethics is that professionals are especially powerful in relation to the users of the services, who then become vulnerable to exploitation, abuse or other forms of poor treatment (Benner et al., 2009; Banks and Gallagher, 2009). Banks and Gallagher (2009) suggest that professionals need to be aware of the power inherent in their role and the vulnerability and dependency of the people. The events at Mid Staffordshire NHS Foundation Trust demonstrate how such vulnerability and dependency can expose patients to abuse and exploitation. For example, patients were left in excrement and soiled clothes for long periods of time; assistance with food and drink was not provided to those patients who needed it; and privacy and dignity were denied, even in death (Francis, 2013: 13).

Conditions That Support Compassionate Nursing

Here I draw on the concept analysis to suggest the real challenge with regard to compassion lies within ourselves and the environment in which we work. I propose that we should consider two conditions which are the most important in delivering compassion in nursing.

Self-compassion

The concept of self-compassion in relation to nursing was studied by Reyes (2012). She describes self-compassion as a state of being which provides an understanding of suffering, leading to compassionate caring. This is supported by Gilbert (2009), who suggests that developing self-kindness and self-compassion helps to create caring and compassionate relationships. The notion that self-compassion results in actions to relieve the suffering of others is not new. It features in Buddhist philosophy (Michie, 2012) and is widely acknowledged in the literature (Cingel, 2009; Gilbert, 2009; Dewar, 2011; Hofmann, Grossman and Hinton, 2011; Youngson, 2012; White, 2013; Boellinghaus, Jones and Hutton, 2014). Gilbert (2009) claims that our ability to feel compassion can be dependent on our ability to tolerate threat or distress. If the delivery of compassionate care is dependent on self-compassion, this must be a requirement of compassionate nursing.

Compassionate Organisations

The culture of the NHS has changed significantly in recent years, moving from the values of the welfare state to a model based on a belief that a competitive, business-focused NHS will lead to improvements in healthcare (Crawford et al., 2013). Conversely, the opposite seems to be true; public dissatisfaction with care and reports of poor care have increased. Misinterpretations in the media have laid the blame with nurses, portraying a lack of concern and compassion within the nursing profession. Increasing the focus on the importance of compassion in the working environment may provide a more appropriate rationale for healthcare organisations (Gilbert, 2009; Youngson, 2012; Crawford et al., 2013). A compassionate environment would promote compassionate care. Concern should focus on the culture of organisations, rather than the behaviours and practices of individuals or professional groups such as nurses. In this context, a compassionate working environment is viewed as a necessary prerequisite for compassionate nursing care (this is discussed further by Ghisoni in Chapter 6).

Consequences

The assumptions made in reports and guidance relating to compassion in nursing suggest that patient outcomes and experience are positive where compassionate nursing is present (The Patient Association, 2009, 2010, 2011, 2012; Parliamentary and Health Service Ombudsman, 2011; Francis, 2013). The views expressed by participants in my research interviews endorse this. Compassion theorists also support this, claiming that when compassion is demonstrated care enhances healing and well-being

(Benner et al., 2009; Chambers and Ryder, 2009; Gilbert, 2009), alleviates distress, and leads to contentment, coping, confidence, satisfaction and empowerment (Burnard, 1997; Gilbert, 2009; Chambers and Ryder, 2009; Youngson, 2012).

Empirical Referents

Despite increasing demands for compassionate nursing care, there has been little research in this area. Studies have demonstrated examples where compassion is absent (Hem and Heggen, 2004) and where it is present (Smith et al., 2010; Dewar, 2011), through observation in practice and the application of purposeful interventions, respectively. Importantly, although compassion is considered to be fundamental to nursing (Dietze and Orb, 2000; Schantz, 2007; Youngson, 2008; Firth-Cozens and Cornwell, 2009; Chambers and Ryder, 2009; Maben et al., 2010), the conclusions from the literature suggest that applying and monitoring compassion in nursing practice is complex (Dietze and Orb, 2000; Hem and Heggen, 2004; Schantz, 2007; Firth-Cozens and Cornwell, 2009; Maben et al., 2010). Furthermore, its application in relation to achieving good patient outcomes and satisfaction remains unclear (Dietze and Orb, 2000; Youngson, 2008; Firth-Cozens and Cornwell, 2009; Maben et al., 2010).

A framework for the implementation of compassionate nursing care in hospital has provided some indication of how it may be applied and monitored (Dewar, 2011). However, this and other theories regarding compassion in nursing (Chambers and Ryder, 2009; Cummings and Bennett, 2012) describe compassionate care through activities and approaches that are concepts or descriptions in their own right, for example competence, communication, caring, collaboration, person-centeredness, empathy, relationships, dignity and so on. I wish to add to this debate by exploring the meaning and significance of compassion in nursing and to make a distinction between what constitutes good nursing care and what might be seen as compassionate care.

It is clear from nationally published stories (The Patients Association, 2009, 2010, 2011, 2012; Parliamentary and Health Service Ombudsman, 2011) and from the emerging findings of my research that the expectations and experiences of individual patients and their families vary immensely, as do the actions required to meet their needs. With this in mind, the act of compassion as a singular concept is difficult to describe. Although good nursing care may include actions and approaches such as empathy, dignity, physical acts of caring and ethical conduct, compassion appears to be an 'enabler' to those actions and behaviours rather than an additional contributory factor. It seems to be the single factor that leads one nurse to act in a way that meets the needs and expectations of the patient, where another does not. In recent years, there has been a move towards promoting compassion within education and performance review. Yet the question remains: 'is compassion something you can teach and is it easy to see?' In my experience of nursing, I have heard experienced nurses attempting to describe what it is that makes a good nurse and have heard the phrase 'You just know when you have a good one', many times. Furthermore, compassion appears to be more than the sum of its parts, which are unique to the patient's situation.

Conclusion and Recommendations

This concept analysis has explored the complex and multifaceted characteristics and conditions for compassion in nursing. The representation of compassion in the literature, reports and policy documents includes some inconsistent descriptions and claims regarding compassionate care, and the word *compassion* is often used interchangeably with other concepts. Crucially, there is little empirical evidence to describe compassion as an essential ingredient of nursing care.

The defining attributes of compassion in regard to nursing have been identified as kindness, empathy, caring, dignity and upholding professional conduct and practice in order to protect people from harm, consider their rights and promote autonomy and beneficence; and recognition of a need for care, with a wish to do something about it (Figure 3.1). These concepts are in themselves complex and have a number of meanings. As such, the meaning and significance of compassion is subject to interpretation. For this reason, it is essential that nurses understand and become conversant with compassion as a concept.

If nurses are to influence patient experience and outcomes through the delivery of compassion, the meaning and significance of compassion in the context of healthcare today must be clarified. Research is needed to ensure that compassion is viewed as an essential component of nursing, integral to the moral, ethical and professional responsibilities that constitute nursing intelligence and expertise. In addition, the conditions required to ensure that compassionate care is possible – that is, promoting compassionate caring environments – must be a priority. This presents an added challenge in the face of the pressures of working within health and social care environments in 2016 and beyond.

Notes

1. 'An Exploration of Compassion in Nursing: The Meaning and Significance of Compassionate Nursing Care for Older People in Hospital', PhD thesis, submission due 2016.
2. Since writing this concept analysis, the NMC code of conduct has been published and states that registered nurses and midwifes must 'treat people with kindness, respect and compassion' (NMC [2015] *The Code: Professional Standards of Practice and Behaviour for Nurses and Midwives*, www.nmc.org.uk/globalassets/sitedocuments/nmc-publications/revised-new-nmc-code.pdf).

References

Alzheimer's Society (2009) *Counting the Cost: Caring for People with Dementia on Hospital Wards* (London: Alzheimer's Society).

Ballatt, J. and P. Campling (2011) *Intelligent Kindness: Reforming the Culture of Healthcare* (London: The Royal College of Psychiatrists).

Banks, S. and A. Gallagher (2009) *Ethics in Professional Life: Virtues for Health and Social Care* (Basingstoke: Palgrave Macmillan).

Benner, P. (1984) *From Novice to Expert: Excellence and Power in Clinical Nursing Practice* (Menlo Park, CA: Addison-Wesley).

Benner, P., C. Tanner and C. Chesla (2009) *Expertise in Nursing Practice: Caring, Clinical Judgment, and Ethics*, 2nd edn (New York: Springer).

Benner, P. and J. Wrubel (1989) *The Primacy of Caring: Stress and Coping in Health and Illness* (Menlo Park, CA: Addison-Wesley Publishing).

Bible Gateway (2011) Luke 10: 25–37: The Parable of the Good Samaritan, www.biblegateway.com/passage/?search=Luke%2010:25-37, accessed 12 March 2014.

Boellinghaus, I., F. W. Jones and J. Hutton (2014) 'The Role of Mindfulness and Loving-Kindness Meditation in Cultivating Self-Compassion and Other-Focused Concern in Healthcare Professionals', *Mindfulness*, 5: 129–38.

Burnard, P. (1997) 'Why Care? Ethical and Spiritual Issues in Caring in Nursing', in G. Brykczynska (ed.) *Caring: The Compassion and Wisdom of Nursing* (London: Arnold), 32–44.

Cambridge English Dictionary (2014) Definition of 'compassion', http://dictionary.cambridge.org/dictionary/british/compassion, accessed 21 January 2014.

Chambers, C. and E. Ryder (2009) *Compassion and Caring in Nursing* (Oxford: Radcliffe).

Chochinov, H. M. (2007) 'Dignity and the Essence of Medicine: The A, B, C, and D of Dignity Conserving Care', *British Medical Journal*, 335(7612): 184–7.

Cingel, M. (2009) 'Compassion and Professional Care: Exploring the Domain', *Nursing Philosophy*, 10: 124–36.

Clegg, S. and S. Rowland (2010) 'Kindness in Pedagogical Practice and Academic Life', *British Journal of Sociology of Education*, 31(6): 719–35.

Corbin, J. and A. Strauss (2008) *Basics of Qualitative Research: Techniques and Procedures for Developing Grounded Theory,* 3rd edn (Thousand Oaks, CA: Sage Publications).

Crawford, P., P. Gilbert, J. Gilbert, C. Gale and K. Harvey (2013) 'The Language of Compassion in Acute Mental Healthcare', *Qualitative Health Research,* 23(6): 719–27.

Cummings, J. and V. Bennett (2012) *Compassion in Practice: Nursing, Midwifery and Care Staff Our Vision and Strategy* (London: DH).

Department of Health (DH) (2008) *High Quality Care for All – NHS Next Stage Review Final Report* (London: DH).

Department of Health (DH) (2009a) *The NHS Constitution for England* (London: The Stationery Office).

Department of Health (2009b) *Prime Minister's Commission on the Future of Nursing and Midwifery* (London: DH).

Department of Health (DH) (2012) *Prime Minister's Challenge on Dementia: Delivering Major Improvements in Dementia Care and Research by 2015,* www. dh.gov.uk/health/2012/03/pm-dementia-challenge, accessed 10 January 2014.

Department of Health (DH) (2013) *Report of the Mid Staffordshire NHS Trust Public Inquiry*, Executive Summary, Francis, R. [QC] (London: The Stationery Office).

Dewar, B. (2011) *Caring about Caring: An Appreciative Inquiry about Compassionate Relationship-Centred Care*, PhD thesis submitted to Edinburgh Napier, Faculty of Health, Life and Social Sciences, School of Nursing, Midwifery and Social Care, October 2011, Edinburgh.

Dewar, B. and R. Mackay (2010) 'Appreciating and Developing Compassionate Care in an Acute Hospital Setting Caring for Older People', *International Journal of Older People Nursing* 5(4): 299–308.

Dietze, E. and A. Orb (2000) 'Compassionate Care: A Moral Dimension of Nursing', *Nursing Inquiry,* 7: 166–74.

Dinkins, C. (2011) 'Ethics: Beyond Patient Care: Practicing Empathy in the Workplace', *Online Journal of Issues in Nursing,* 16(2), www.nursingworld. org/MainMenuCategories/ANAMarketplace/ANAPeriodicals/OJIN/Columns/ Ethics/Empathy-in-the-Workplace.html, accessed 16 April 2014.

Ferrell, B. F. and N. Coyle (2008) *The Nature of Suffering and the Goals of Nursing* (Oxford: Oxford University Press).

Firth-Cozens, J. and J. Cornwell (2009) *The Point of Care: Enabling Compassion in Acute Hospital Settings* (London: The King's Fund).

Forrest, C. (2011) 'Nursing with Kindness and Compassion', *Independent Nurse,* 10: 38, www.magonlinelibrary.com.libaccess.hud.ac.uk/, accessed 12 March 2014. doi/full/10.12968/indn.2011.17.10.

Gilbert, P. (2010) *The Compassionate Mind: A New Approach to Life's Challenges* (London: Constable).

Hem, M. H. and M. Heggen (2004) 'Is Compassion Essential for Nursing Practice?', *Contemporary Nurse,* 17: 19–31.

Hofmann, S. G., P. Grossman and D. E. Hinton (2011) 'Loving-Kindness and Compassion Meditation: Potential for Psychological Interventions', *Clinical Psychology Review,* 31: 1126–32.

Johnson, M., C. Haigh and N. Yates-Bolton (2007) 'Valuing of Altruism and Honesty in Nursing Students: A Two-Decade Replication Study', *Journal of Advanced Nursing*, 57(4): 366–74.

Maben, J., J. Cornwell and K. Sweeney (2010) 'In Praise of Compassion', *Journal of Research in Nursing*, 15: 9–13.

Michie, D. (2012) *Enlightenment to Go: Shantideva and the Power of Compassion to Transform Your Life* (Boston: Wisdom Publications).

Miller, B. F. and C. B. Keane (1989) *Encyclopedia and Dictionary of Medicine, Nursing and Applied Health* (Philadelphia: Saunders).

Milton, C. L. (2013) 'Suffering', *Nursing Science Quarterly*, 26(3): 226–8.

National Health Service (NHS) Confederation (2008) *Compassion In Healthcare: The Missing Dimension of Healthcare Reform? Futures Debate*, paper, 2 May, www.nhsconfed.org/Publications/Documents/compassion, accessed 14 March 2014.

NHS Confederation, Age UK and Local Government Association (2012) *Delivering Dignity: Securing Dignity in Care for Older People in Hospitals and Care Homes. A Report for Consultation*, www.nhsconfed.org/Documents/Delivering_Dignity.pdf, accessed 12 March 2014.

Nursing and Midwifery Council (NMC) (2015) *The Code: Professional Standards of Practice and Behaviour for Nurses and Midwives*, ww.nmc.org.uk/globalassets/sitedocuments/nmc-publications/revised-new-nmc-code.pdf.

Nursing and Midwifery Council (NMC) (2010) *Standards for Pre-registration Nursing Education*, http://standards.nmc-uk.org/PublishedDocuments/Standardsforpre-registrationnursingeducation2016082010.pdf, accessed 12 March 2014.

Nursing and Midwifery Council (NMC) (2008) 'The Code: Standards of Conduct, Performance and Ethics for Nurses and Midwives', www.nmc-uk.org/Publications/Standards/The-code, accessed 12 March 2014.

Parliamentary and Health Service Ombudsman (2011) *Care and Compassion? Report of the Health Service Ombudsman on Ten Investigations into NHS Care of Older People.* (London: The Stationery Office).

Reyes, D. (2012) 'Self-Compassion: A Concept Analysis', *Journal of Holistic Nursing*, 30(2): 81–89.

Royal College of Nursing (RCN) (2014) 'Key Concepts of Person-Centred Care', www.rcn.org.uk/development/practice/cpd_online_learning/dignity_in_health_care/person-centred_care, accessed 26 May 2014.

Royal College of Nursing (RCN) (2010) 'Gordon Brown Addresses RCN Congress', www.rcn.org.uk/newsevents/congress/2010/monday, accessed 10 January 2014.

Royal College of Nursing (RCN) (2009) 'RCN Dignity Campaign', www.rcn.org.uk/__data/assets/pdf_file/0003/265530/003291.pdf, accessed 12 March 2014.

Royal College of Nursing (RCN) (2008) 'RCN Definition of "dignity"', www.rcn.org.uk/__data/assets/pdf_file/0003/191730/003298.pdf, accessed 12 March 2014.

Sayer, A. (2005) *The Moral Significance of Class* (Cambridge: Cambridge University Press).

Schantz, M. L. (2007) 'Compassion: A Concept Analysis', *Nursing Forum* 42(2): 48–55.

Smith, S., B. Dewar and S. Pullin (2010) 'Relationship Outcomes Focused on Compassionate Care for Older People within Inpatient Care Settings', *International Journal of Older People Nursing*, 5(2): 128–36.

Straughair, C. (2012) 'Exploring Compassion: Implications for Contemporary Nursing, Part 2', *British Journal of Nursing*, 21(4): 239–44.

Tadd, W., A. Hillman, S. Calnan, M. Calnan, T. Bayer and S. Read (2011) *Dignity in Practice: An Exploration of the Care of Older Adults in Acute NHS Trusts* (London: DH).

The Patients Association (2012) 'Stories from the Present: Lessons for the Future', www.patients-association.org.uk, accessed 10 January 2014.

The Patient's Association (2011) 'We've Been Listening, Have You Been Learning?', www.patients-association.org.uk, accessed 10 January 2014.

The Patient's Association (2010) 'Listen to Patients, Speak up for Change', www.patients-association.org.uk/dbimgs/listentopatients,speakupforchange, accessed 10 January 2014.

The Patient's Association (2009) 'Patients Not Numbers, People Not Statistics', www.patients-association.org.uk/News/307, accessed 10 January 2014.

Walker, L. O. and K. C. Avant (2011) *Strategies for Theory Constructing in Nursing* (Upper Saddle River, NJ: Prentice Hall).

White, L. (2013) Mindfulness in Nursing: An Evolutionary Concept Analysis', *Journal of Advanced Nursing*, www.wileyonlinelibrary.com/journal/jan, accessed 15 May 2014.

Wiseman, T. (1996) 'A Concept Analysis of Empathy', *Journal of Advanced Nursing*, 23: 1163–7.

Youngson, R. (2012) *Time to Care: How to Love Your Patients and Your Job* (New Zealand: Rebelheart).

Youngson, R. (2008) *Compassion in Healthcare: The Missing Dimension of Healthcare Reform?* (London: NHS Confederation).

4

What Compassion Means: The Person and Family Perspective

Georgina Craig

Introduction

The purpose of The Experience Led Commissioning (ELC) Programme is to support National Health Service (NHS) commissioners – the clinicians and managers who buy NHS services and determine the outcomes that get measured – to walk in the shoes of the people, families and front-line teams who deliver care. Using mainly semi-structured interview techniques and co-design approaches that draw on experience-based co-design (Bate and Robert, 2012), we collect stories and identify the critical emotional touch points in the care journey. Then we aggregate, interpret and make sense of these stories so that commissioners have actionable insights to inform their metrics, planning and contracting processes. We also work closely with the charity Healthtalk (www.healthtalk.org). The qualitative data they use provides ELC with a benchmark for the local stories we hear. This helps us to explore both the differences and similarities across communities.

In this chapter, we present insights from patients with dementia and stroke, which explore their experiences of care. This chapter differs from others in the book in that it is not examining research or theory. Rather, it seeks to illustrate, through people's lived experiences, how theory translates into real life. For us, stories – or narratives as they are sometimes called – are the source from which we draw evidence about what matters to people. We define narratives as the first-person descriptions of people's lived experiences, told from their perspective and in their own words. Being true to what people tell us is essential to the practice of ELC.

Policy Context

The NHS Outcomes Framework (NHS England, 2014) put delivering outcomes related to experience on an equal footing with clinical outcomes within the NHS commissioning system. NHS performance management

Experience is NOT satisfaction
(Betty, 75 years old, on Medicine for the Elderly ward)

The other thing I didn't raise and I should have done because it does annoy me intensely, the time you have to wait for a bedpan. ... elderly people can't wait, if we want a bedpan it's because we need it now. I just said to one of them, 'I need a bedpan please.' And it was so long bringing it out it was too late. It's a very embarrassing subject, although they don't make anything of it, they just say, Oh well, it can't be helped if you're not well.' And I thought, 'Well, if only you'd brought the bedpan you wouldn't have to strip the bed and I wouldn't be so embarrassed."

Betty's patient survey

Q: overall, did you feel you were treated with respect and dignity while you were in hospital?

Yes, always

Q: overall, how do you rate the care you received?

Excellent

Figure 4.1 Patient satisfaction is not experience of care.
Source: Maben J, Peccei R, Adams M, Robert G, Richardson A, Murrells T and Morrow E. Patients' experiences of care and the influence of staff motivation, affect and wellbeing. Phase II case studies: Annexe to final report. NIHR Service Delivery and Organisation programme; 2012: pages 17–18.

relies mainly on quantitative measures such as patient satisfaction surveys and Friends and Family Test (NHS England, 2014) (see also Chapter 1 for a discussion of related policy issues). As research shows (Maben et al., 2012), these 'black-and-white' measurement tools can be misleading and mask a very different story (see Figure 4.1 for example).

To get a richer picture of people's experiences, we need to dig a little deeper into the stories behind the numbers. This chapter introduces a framework to help the reader to do just that. Developed through a collaboration between academics from nursing and health experience research (Kitson et al., 2013), it seeks to understand how patients experience the fundamentals of care, including elimination, personal hygiene and eating – and how the way nurses behave and manage care impacts on people's feelings of dignity and respect.

Informed by secondary thematic reanalysis of primary narrative interview data collected from stroke survivors about their inpatient care (Kitson et al., 2013), researchers produced a three-dimensional framework for understanding how people experience care. We have applied this same framework here to help the reader explore and make sense of how people and families experience care as compassionate – both in hospital and community settings – so that nurses can reflect on and start to recognise the '3D' nature of the care experience – and how the three different elements come together and create both positive and negative stories in people's minds.

To illustrate this interplay, we draw on the experiences of the following people:

> Stroke survivors with severe impairment and prolonged experience of inpatient care.

> People who live with two or more long-term health conditions, including dementia.

The stroke stories come from the original secondary thematic analysis (Kitson et al., 2013). Dementia stories are drawn from the www .healthtalk.org archive. Stories of living with long-term health can be found in the archives of The Experience Led Commissioning Programme (www.experienceledcare.co.uk) and were generated when we or the local teams we work with talked to people and families about their experiences of care.

Illustrated with extracts from the patient stories, this chapter looks at care through three lenses:

1. Physical

2. Psychosocial

3. Relational.

The integration of the physical and psychosocial elements of care is mediated by relationships with caring professionals. The three dimensions are inextricably bound in the minds of people and families and rarely untangle. If an element is missing at any stage, people experience distress and a lack of compassion. This means that to create a compassionate experience, nurses need to respond to all three elements. A three-dimensional understanding of experience is more accurate than more hierarchical or linear models. This 3D model also fits with what we hear from the people and families we talk to and work with.

Each element is now considered in turn:

Physical

Needing help with intimate physical tasks is a fundamental shift for most people. Reconciling their new need for help has a profound impact on the person. In this section, we cover a number of the key elements of physical care from the framework and illustrate that nurses perform acts of physical care impacts on compassion. The stories demonstrate that the quality of support and care people receive with their physical needs has a psychosocial and emotional impact. Kitson et al. (2013) conclude that good physical care builds confidence and accelerates recovery, whereas de-humanised physical care results in humiliation, distress and compromises dignity. They also argue that positive experiences are less memorable and that the distressing experiences endure (Kitson et al., 2013). This reinforces the importance of delivering a positive experience for patients, because poor care has long-lasting negative effects.

Mobility. Reduced mobility has a significant impact on mental well-being:

> My (young) daughter has come out with a couple of things that have been said. She doesn't say very much, but one of the things she said was 'When the surgeons cut my Dad's leg off, they also took away all his happiness.'

When a health condition reduces mobility and the person has to rely on others, the way a nurse delivers care can create or destroy compassion:

> [T]here would, come a time when you were taken to the toilet or bathroom, and there were various devices to try and swizzle you into the bath from a standing position. And there was a way of achieving this with some care and diligence and equally a way of doing it with no interest, indeed disinterest frankly, and a wholesale lack of caring.

In community settings, losing mobility can also be life changing for people. Without access to the right home modifications, intimate personal care can become extremely difficult. This also destroys dignity and independence:

> Oh it was a pain. I used to wash at the sink in the kitchen. I used to go to the toilet. I'd have to put my splints on to go to the toilet. I couldn't get upstairs. I used to have to put my splints on to go to the toilet, but before that they had – before that they gave me a commode, just a cheap commode really – not like nothing you'd get in the hospital because it was just what they send you

home with if you like – which was really not hygienic. Because if I'd got to go to the toilet, I have to go in the kitchen because of my daughter, and I complained about it. I said, 'Because it's a food prep area. And you're making me go to toilet in my kitchen.' I said, 'How unhygienic is that?' I said, 'You have it. You do it.' So they got the toilet done for me.

If care staff can show empathy for people and support them in accessing home modifications and equipment that maintain independence, they will be contributing to compassionate care.

Elimination. Stroke survivors describe the anxiety fuelled by the unfamiliar mechanics of equipment used to support elimination. When no one explains what is going on, they experience a loss of dignity, which affects their emotional well-being:

I remember the first time I went to the loo in the stroke unit, I was taken in a sort of cage affair. You're strapped into a device alongside the bed, flat, and you're then put upright on this device and you're wheeled to the toilet and you're gradually lowered over the loo by, from this, this device ... It's very, very – what's the word? Intrusive, I suppose, and [it] made me very, very depressed.

Explaining how equipment works and being sensitive and reassuring about the process create compassion.

Eating and drinking. Loss of mobility can also have an impact on eating and drinking in stroke survivors:

Another big problem is food when you're newly paralysed, is eating, because it's difficult to eat with only one arm, and you can't cut food up, and hospital food tends to come in little plastic wrappers that I couldn't open with butter to spread on biscuits that I couldn't spread because you need two hands.

Hospital food – especially pureed food – can be unappetising:

I think the worst part at that time was probably being on liquid diet; I had to have all my food pureed, which was revolting.

Staff do not always recognise that people need support with eating and drinking. People often feel left to their own devices. Sometimes food is left out of reach or people receive no assistance with eating. The Care Quality

Commission (CQC) investigated this issue in hospitals (CQC, 2011) and care homes (CQC, 2012) and found 12 per cent of hospitals and 17 per cent of care homes were not meeting standards for nutrition.

When supporting patients with dementia, nurses should recognise that they may need to remind the person to eat or show him or her how to eat. Addressing this requires patience and empathy. Empathy has been defined as the intellectual and emotional awareness and understanding of another person's thoughts, feelings and behaviour, even those that are distressing and disturbing (Miller and Keane, 1989). One family carer describes how she managed to teach her mother to eat again with support from the district nurse:

> No I don't think you should force drink, I don't think you should force anything down ... I think it's a question of finding out what the person understands, because my mother could understand a drink in a cup ... So I then said to the home, 'Could you put her soup in the mug because she can understand the mug, she can't understand the bowl and the spoon?'... The district nurse, being the professional that she is, said that if your mother goes to a table with others and sees other people eating, she may try and copy, which in fact in time to come she did ... I'm not a professional I don't know, but I would say that if they stop eating, try and offer them things that they understand ... so I think it's much better to, by trial and error, find out the things that the sufferer is happy to take.

Personal cleansing and dressing. People experienced emotional anxiety and embarrassment when they were unable to wash independently. Loss of personal standards of hygiene, feeling unclean, smelling, having unkempt hair or not wearing their own clothes was humiliating. The emotional impact is not always recognised by nursing staff:

> The jobs which nurses used to do like pressure care, tidying the bed at night, bringing you a wash bowl, your mouth wash, if you have dentures you want to clean them, or if not, after a meal you want to clean your teeth and rinse; that was very much lacking I must say, and that did upset me.

Helping patients take control of washing and dressing can be an important turning point signalling a return to independence and a sense of self. Working together and setting small goals to advance towards is an important element of compassionate care:

> They brought a – a thing of water to the bed and a flannel and some soap and the first day I washed myself in bed and I cleaned my teeth after about 4 days. It was absolutely wonderful, and that was a turning point.

Medication. Medication is an important part of most people's experience of care, particularly those with long-term conditions. For example, stroke survivors discuss the importance of being aware of and understanding the side effects of medication so they feel in control of the tablets that others are administering to them:

> I'm somebody who really rather shied away from medication before; I wouldn't even take an aspirin for the flu. I had to learn how to swallow pills in – in numbers …

For people with dementia and their families, the issues are quite different. Medication is often ineffective in halting the progression of dementia. Many family carers feel this is because it is prescribed too late because the diagnosis is not made early enough. People with dementia are usually taking medication for other long-term health issues too.

Prompting people to remember to take medication is something that family carers often do, and a role that nurses may need to take over when the family carer is not present. Sometimes people with dementia can experience problems swallowing. They may also refuse to take medication because they no longer recognise that taking medication is part of their daily routine. Understanding what lies behind apparent refusal and working with the person with dementia helps build compassion.

Psychosocial

The psychosocial element of care involves recognition that health conditions and experiences of care affect people's sense of identity, existence and self-worth. For instance, how does managing their feelings of personal disgust and humiliation at having to depend on another person to undertake acts of personal care affect them? And equally, how do nurses as caregivers – or family carers – manage the disgust and humiliation they may experience on their own and the person's behalf when they have to provide intimate care? As we have seen, people do not distinguish between the physical and psychosocial elements of the care experience. This means that the physical act of caring always has a psychosocial impact. The psychosocial elements are examined below.

Dignity. People do not talk about compassion in their stories; rather, they discuss the importance of dignity and how nurses do or do not support them to preserve dignity. As noted earlier, people tell us that these memories remain vivid despite the passage of time:

I felt as if I was wetting myself and that was really, really humiliating. I really felt – I felt the pits, you know, and it was before my wife came in and she said, 'What's wrong with you?' and I didn't explain, you know. I said, 'It's just this catheter', you know. But that must have been the lowest, lowest point I was, so I felt – I felt I was wetting myself, you know. There was nothing I could do. I had been to the toilet before I went. I knew I was going to need – you know, and I felt so humiliated. I really felt so low, it was ridiculous. It really, really was. That was a low point. The lowest point I would think, I would think possibly the lowest point.

I got very distressed because obviously it had gone on all over my nighty and on the bed and I cried; I really, really cried just out of – I felt really degraded because I'd been left to do it on my own and because I couldn't get up and go to the loo, and it was so frightening not to have the control of your body.

Needing help with intimate personal care can lead to loss of self-esteem, self-confidence, independence and motivation. People talk of their physical body becoming uncoupled from their sense of self:

Things like personal hygiene – I mean, is – your – one's dignity is absolutely stripped, it is; it is like being a baby with an adult mind [eh] in a rather badly run boarding school actually.

People feel they struggle alone to protect their dignity in a hospital that feels like a battlefield. This sense of isolation is exacerbated when they feel unable to connect with their care team on a human level:

I just thought I don't want them helping me because there was no one on the ward that I had any regard or respect for.

Communication and education. Stroke survivors often struggle to communicate:

Talking was very difficult for me in those first few days. I could talk, but it actually sounded as if I was permanently drunk, I suppose. It was very slurred, and I found it difficult to get the words out; you find it very difficult to absorb things.

Caring, approachable staff have a positive impact on patients' experience:

But it's just being approachable enough I would say for health care professionals, that people actually feel that because sometimes it's very difficult to ask for very personal help if it's something you're not used to asking for, even though it's something you obviously need. It's difficult to actually ask for it. Because I don't feel like I'm a survivor of a stroke; I feel I'm struggling – I'm struggling with the stroke, but I don't think I want to be called a struggler either. Just a person. I think sometimes a person is not seen.

In dementia, the challenge of communication is different. One woman with dementia describes how communication feels for her:

It's also an embarrassment at times. You know, in conversation with people you suddenly realise that 'Oh, heck, I think we've had this conversation before', but I can't remember. Or we've been somewhere ... I can't remember to tell [my husband] what it's all about. It's very, very annoying. I have to look at the programme and say, 'Oh, yes, that's right. It was.' That's, you know, it impinges on your communicating with people, really, because if it's not coming smoothly, you tend to shut up. And I don't want to do that. They might, but I don't ... There's also a worry that you're going to become a very boring person because you can't maintain conversation.

Family carers experience the distress of watching their loved ones lose their words:

Conversation with neighbours, with friends and relatives, changed, because now I realise that she was losing her vocabulary, losing the understanding of words and therefore finding it difficult to have a conversation. After the diagnosis, that became easier to understand and accept, and at least I could then explain to the people what was happening with my wife and ... the behavioural changes that were taking place.

For those in the later stages of dementia, touch is an important form of communication – and one that professionals may shy away from or misinterpret. For example, one carer describes her concern when care staff objected to her husband's desire to touch them. Since he could no longer speak, physical contact was his only means of communicating. She felt care staff should not be afraid to touch people with dementia or be touched by them:

And I do think that the best way of communicating with people in the middle to late phases of dementia is through touch, through holding their hand, through smiling, to convey [...] information in ways other than words which they understand and [to] which they can [...] respond, if they wish to. Obviously some people don't want to be touched; I understand that, but I think the staff at least should give the person with dementia the benefit of the doubt if they want to be touched. And if they want to touch them, then that is a[n] human act of kindness and has no sexual or other meaning to it. Mostly!

Privacy and respecting choice. People describe privacy in hospital in terms of place and space on the ward, feeling they are in a safe place and being able to move around. They also talk about maintaining personal modesty, integrity and balancing their need for privacy with not becoming isolated. When we have done Experience Led Commissioning work with residents in care homes, they talk similarly about their space. For instance, having somewhere to entertain relatives really matters to them. For most people, choice means feeling involved and in control of one's treatment and therapy. Recognising a person's right to refuse treatment is part of compassion:

> They have wanted for a long time for me to be on warfarin, and I have refused, and it's not only because it's rat poison, though of course that doesn't help. I've said from the start I didn't want to be because I'm very clumsy. I'm always fall-ing over and banging into things, and therefore using warfarin for me, would not be a good idea. I didn't like the idea of constant blood tests and [sighs] – well, I'm prepared to take the risk.

Other choices that matter – particularly in hospital settings – include showers or baths, and male carers rather than female carers. Working together as a nursing team to respond to these choices enhances com-passion. The issues surrounding choice are different for people with dementia. For example, in many cases they cannot cope with questions. Communication needs to support them to exercise choice in a different way:

> And another thing is the joy – one of the conveniences of Alzheimer's is if you say 'Would you like a drink?' and she'll say 'No I don't want to take it,' and you'll put it down. You can actually say it as if you're saying it afresh a couple of minutes later. Sadly the carers at the home where mum is, don't all realise that, they'll go 'You must take this [...] because it's going to make you better,' and she's lost her powers of reason now so it's better to just put it down again and say, talk about something else or sit there for a bit longer. And 'Oh would you like a drink?' 'Oh thank you.' And she might take a sip and say 'Oh I don't like that very much.' 'Oh well put it down and have it later' you know.

Family carers often continue with activities the person enjoyed before the onset of his or her condition:

> I've tried to keep up the kind of standards which [my wife] would have insisted on when she was in full health ... I try to make meal times as pleasurable as I

possibly can. I try to ensure that we set the table as nicely as we can; we have wine to drink with our meals. I usually have some of her favourite music playing in the background. So we try to make an occasion of most of the meals that we have.

It is important when caring for people that nurses involve and work with family carers and ask them about what matters and help them to maintain the standards that they feel preserves their loved one's dignity. This creates compassion. This framework suggests that nurses who deliver physical care in ways that identify and preserve dignity will be practising compassionate care.

Relational

When people are unable to connect on a human level with their caregiver – in particular when they require help with elimination, personal dressing and cleansing – they can experience humiliation and loss. Taking a structured approach to building relationships by setting shared goals and displaying empathy is key within the framework.

Personal goal setting. People start to lose hope when they cannot do the simple tasks they used to enjoy:

> I remember one day – day, I said, 'I'm going to try doing a crossword puzzle' and I got – I got the pencil out and had the answer but I couldn't put the letters in the square box for the crossword puzzle and that really got me, you know, I was feeling quite depressed.

Setting small, personalised goals together builds a sense of partnership and thus positive relationships between staff and people:

> It's, you know – and it was the goal-setting was really – we have a sheet there we – we fill in from week to week of what we want to achieve next week, fortnight, 3 weeks down the line and you work towards that and it – it kind of takes your mind off your illness or, – or your injury, as far as I'm concerned.

Patients identified occupational and physiotherapists as being especially skilled in this area:

> [T]hey seemed to do it in such a way that you – you feel you're making progress, you feel you're making a step forward, you know. And you feel you're actually, 'Yeah, I'm getting better.'

Nurses who build shared goal setting into their practice create compassion.

Empathy. Empathy is the ability to understand another person's condition from their perspective, placing yourself in their shoes and feeling what they are feeling. Accounts of empathetic care are rare amongst stroke survivors.

> They were great. They give you the respect. They'll stand outside the room while you get your underwear on or off or whatever.

> Yes, there are good nurses where they will relax and first they will find out whether – are you feeling thirsty, are you feeling tired, Very simple things.

A mixed picture is more common:

> For every caring, intelligent, supportive member of hospital staff ... for every one of those who is good and supportive at their – at their profession, I would also say that there's probably an equal number who don't take the same pride in their job and who don't care very much about the feeling, sensitivities and ultimate condition of their patients ...

> Health professionals are good as far as assessment or medication, its effect and their knowledge about how the body works, they are very good at it. Emotions – and they only read from books and I don't think they are so much good. They might not have that much experience to talk to you because they don't have time.

Empathy and forming relationships with those with dementia is particularly important. When empathy happens, it can be life changing for the family:

> as if they were part of the family and she was part of their family and it was the most normal thing that they were coming in here. They would talk about their children, or what they'd done at the weekend. Just friendly, not patronising. Relaxed – and never really giving the impression that there were probably many other people who they'd got to do the same thing for before they clocked off ... Yes, they really seemed not just to be doing a caring role, but to actually care. And to have to capacity to rally somebody who may not want to do what they wanted to do in the time allotted which is another skill really.

People often tell us that relationships matter most. Working with people on personal goals from a position of empathy cements positive relationships. Every nurse can incorporate goal setting into his or her clinical practice and remain curious about people's experiences. Although experiences of lost dignity endure, so do positive memories of the supportive relationships people and families forge with their caregivers. Nurses have opportunities every day to connect with people and create those memories.

Of course, it is impossible for caregivers to know exactly what it is like to be the person until perhaps they experience illness themselves. Often when this happens, health professionals become vocal advocates for change in the way care is delivered. Two recent inspirational stories illustrate the power of clinicians' personal experience on compassionate care.

1. Dr Ann McPherson was a general practitioner who was diagnosed with cancer and could not find out what it is like to live with cancer on a human level. As a result, she co-founded the Database of Individual Patient Experiences (DIPEx) to provide resources to enable people, families and health professionals to understand the lived experiences of health conditions by watching video clips of people talking about their experiences. The website healthtalk.org now covers over 70 health conditions and provides a wealth of insights for curious professionals who want to 'walk in the shoes' of people and families. Ann died in 2011, although her legacy lives on.

2. Kate Granger, @GrangerKate, kick-started the Twitter campaign #hellomynameis after her experiences of hospital care:

> I'm a doctor, but also a terminally ill cancer patient. During a hospital stay, I made the stark observation that many staff looking after me did not introduce themselves before delivering care. This felt wrong, so encouraged and supported by my husband, we decided to start a campaign and remind healthcare staff about the importance of introductions in the delivery of care. I firmly believe that it is not just about knowing someone's name, but it runs much deeper. It is about making a human connection; beginning a therapeutic relationship and building trust. In my mind, it is the first rung on the ladder to providing compassionate care.

Of course, introducing yourself when you meet someone is a social norm and key to establishing rapport and trust, especially before performing an intimate care task. Yet it took Kate's campaign for the NHS to notice that caregivers were performing intimate care tasks every day – and saying nothing.

Conclusion

Kitson et al. (2013) pose a number of challenging questions with regard to compassion.

> If we paid more attention to maintaining the integrity of self during the predictable assault of the disease ... would patients survive more intact? What are the psychological scars that remain when 'dignity has been repeatedly stripped away' each time a person needs to ask for help to go to the toilet and has a humiliating experience? (Kitson et al., 2013: 402)

People's stories challenge us to remember that simple things really matter. Always introducing oneself and performing physical care in a way that preserves self and dignity is not about doing more work. It is more about how we do the work we do. By remaining curious about their experiences and recognising that talking with people and families about how they feel is an essential part of care, nurses can start to notice the small improvements that make a big difference to people's recovery and well-being.

I hope that in considering the material in this chapter, you can identify simple changes that will build compassionate care and positive memories for people and families. Accessing the web resources in this chapter also provides nurses with an opportunity to hear about patients' experiences so that they can continue to develop their skills in delivering compassionate care that is so valued by patients and their families.

References

Bate, P. and G. Robert (2012) 'Experience-Based Design: From Redesigning the System Around the Patient to Co-designing Services with the Patient', *Quality and Safety in Health Care*, 15(5): 307–10.

Care Quality Commission (CQC) (2011) *Dignity and Nutrition Inspection Programme. National Review.* Care Quality Commission.

Care Quality Commission (CQC) (2012) *Time to Listen in Care Home. Dignity and Nutrition Inspection Programme.* Care Quality Commission.

Kitson, A. C. Dow, J. D. Calabrese, L. Locock and A. Muntlin Athlin (2013) 'Stroke Survivors' Experiences of the Fundamentals of Care: A Qualitative Analysis', *International Journal of Nursing Studies*, 50: 392–403.

Maben, J., R. Peccei, M. Adams, G. Robert, A. Richardson, T. Murrells and E. Morrow (2012) *Patients' Experiences of Care and the Influence of Staff Motivation, Affect and Wellbeing. Phase II Case Studies: Annexe to Final Report.* NIHR Service Delivery and Organisation Programme: 17–18.

Miller, B. F. and C. B. Keane (1989) *Encyclopedia and Dictionary of Medicine, Nursing and Applied Health* (Philadelphia: Saunders).

NHS England (2014) *The NHS Outcomes Framework 2015 to 2016*, Department of Health, www.gov.uk/government/publications/nhs-outcomes-framework-2015-to-2016, accessed 10 March 2016.

Acknowledgements

Thank you to all those who shared their stories to help us learn and improve. I would also like to thank Professor Alison Kitson, University of Adelaide, Professor Louise Locock, University of Oxford, and Luís Carrasqueiro from www.healthtalk.org as well as Rachel Sandford from The Experience Led Commissioning Programme for their help and support in preparing this chapter.

5

Healthcare Culture and Intelligent Kindness in Practice

John Ballatt

Introduction

It is rather sad that so much attention must be given to trying to 'restore' compassion to the work of healthcare staff. One of the main reasons is, of course, the frightening abuse and neglect in well-publicised 'scandals' such as Mid Staffordshire and Winterbourne View (NHS England, 2014). Regular, less notorious reports suggest that such failures are even more widespread, which is very troubling, but the debate about what to do about it is almost as alarming. Healthcare staff *must*, the world asserts, be compassionate; job descriptions are modified to say so; policies and guidance make it the rule; people must blow the whistle on failures of compassion; boards must not allow other priorities to intrude; 'organisational cultures' must be transformed (Francis, 2010; DH, 2012a; DH, 2012b).

But why alarming? Well, first, because so little attention is being given in the 'public debate' to the widespread quality and success of the NHS, combined with an increased denigration of the staff who work in it and a concomitant serious risk to their morale. Second, there is little curiosity about what compassion, especially in healthcare, actually entails. How does it work? How is it nourished? What does it involve for staff? Why is it hard to sustain? And finally, because the language of the drive for compassion is so frequently full of 'musts', 'prescriptions', 'duties' and 'specifications', attempts to 'manage' it in this way can actually prevent it being provided.

There is a clue to the problem in the way the discussion so frequently ends up with nursing. As if nurses should 'do' the compassion for the rest of the system as an add-on, or a side issue. Of course, nurses as well as healthcare assistants should work compassionately – and because they are the people who spend the most time with patients, their work offers the greatest opportunity to connect humanely with them. But focusing solely on nursing can distract us from the fact that the whole system needs to foster and sustain compassion; all people working in health and social care need to understand how their work might communicate, help or hinder compassion, and everyone needs the support of the system around them to work compassionately. A healthcare service is a complicated web of relationships – at team, departmental and organisational levels. The quality of these relationships is what determines whether the work is done compassionately and effectively, or not. The purpose of this chapter is to examine how such relationships can be fostered and maintained.

The Psychological Environment

When a nurse on the way through a ward notices that a patient is in distress and diverts from what he or she was doing to help, this is, of course, partly because of the nurse's personal qualities – attentiveness, concern, empathy and so on. However, in the busy, repetitive and routinised setting of a ward, 'noticing', and the associated response, are at least as much the result of the way people work together as a team and the way in which the team and its relationships are managed in the wider organisation. The kind of attention staff give to patients, the humanity and generosity with which they carry out their tasks, is a product of their experience of working with their colleagues and the way in which their work is thought about, organised, supported and managed. 'Putting the patient first' or 'seeing the person in the patient' is not so much the product of a job description or a procedure, as of the quality of the *psychological environment* in which staff work.

This reality has led to much talk of 'getting the culture right', and, of course, that is vital. It is important, though, to understand what this means. Too often, it is interpreted narrowly – we must recruit people with the right attitudes, and we must instruct them in, or remind them of, or inspire them with 'values', the importance of compassion, of person-centred care, of a 'duty of candour' (Francis, 2013) when things go wrong. Culture, though, is actually the expression of how *all* the ingredients and processes in a system interact and of what they draw out, or promote, in the people who work in it. A useful metaphor here is to regard organisational culture as being like an 'ecosystem' in which we are trying to cultivate a crop. The way all the factors in agriculture – light, soil, seeds, rainfall, pests and fertilisers – interact and the way in which they are tended determine the quality of that crop or, in this case, the quality of care.

Whether as healthcare assistants, nurses, doctors or managers, we all need to understand what working together in a 'healthy relational system' means, what such a system looks like when it is there, what helps and hinders it and how our own behaviour influences it. Compassion is one of the things that such a healthy system can nourish and sustain; just as important, however, are imagination, intelligence and readiness to act. The term used most frequently by patients to describe positive experience of care and treatment is *kindness* (see patientopinion.org.uk, for example). The word *compassion* is used far less frequently. Perhaps this is because compassion can focus too much on individuals' feelings about and responses to suffering, whereas kindness suggests both an individual and a collective focus on recognising each other as people – including, but not limited to, responding to 'needs' and 'suffering'.

At the core of compassion, and of a healthy healthcare system, is *kinship*. This idea captures a sense of the recognition that we are of the same *family, kind* or *lineage* as our colleagues and patients. Whatever our differences, we are bound together, and our collective well-being depends on our behaving as *kin* – being *kind* to each other, looking out for each other, combining our efforts for the general good. When we recognise people as *kin*, we are moved to such kindness, to pay attention to what is happening to each other, to act to help or cooperate, to connect and build relationships. The NHS is one of the world's most ambitious (and successful) embodiments of kinship – a reality that requires constant recognition and that means that the system needs the *right kind of nurture*.

A *culture* or a relational system which can nourish such kinship is illustrated in Figure 5.1.

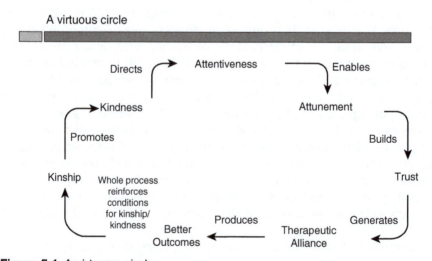

Figure 5.1 A virtuous circle.
Source: Adapted from Ballatt and Campling, 2011.

A Virtuous Circle

In this 'virtuous circle', a recognition of *kinship* promotes in us an attitude of *kindness* – an inclination to consider others' needs and a readiness to respond generously, compassionately and helpfully. As a result, just as a parent responding to an infant, we become *attentive* to others, applying our senses, imagination, empathy and intelligence to what is happening to them, and acting accordingly. This attentiveness leads to *attunement* – we enter a relationship of responsive understanding of another's situation. Experience of an attuned relationship breeds *trust* – which leads to reduced anxiety, to openness, communication and cooperation. Patients who trust their clinicians tend to share more, to listen more and 'cooperate' with their treatment. This sense of trust in turn builds a *therapeutic alliance*, in which both parties are committed to and working together towards improvement. As a result, we achieve *positive outcomes* (not just positive experience, but relief of suffering *and* treatment outcomes). Experience of this 'process' has a reinforcing effect on those involved, promoting a stronger and increasingly positive sense of kinship, which in turn promotes even more inclination to kindness. The whole virtuous circle reduces anxiety and provides a positive sense of common purpose. The connections around the circle, of course, are as important in relationships between colleagues as they are for direct work with patients. Indeed, without them, compassionate care is fragile, sometimes impossible.

This virtuous circle captures what attachment theorists such as John Bowlby have discussed in terms of how early relationships nurture, or fail to nurture, healthy, secure and nourishing ways or habits of relating to others (Bowlby, 1999). The quality of attention, concern, responsiveness and nurture experienced by the infant powerfully influences the growing human being's ability to connect positively with others (Holmes, 1993). Research into psychological therapies has demonstrated that the effectiveness of the therapy depends at least as much on the quality of the trusting relationship with the therapist as on the model of therapy being delivered (Cooper, 2008). There is evidence that wounds heal more slowly when the patient's anxiety is not attended to (Weinman et al., 2008; Cole-King and Harding, 2001). It has been found that patients treated in Accident and Emergency departments who are responded to with 'compassionate care' make fewer return visits and are more satisfied (Rendelmeir, Molin and Tibshirani, 1995). As well as this growing evidence to support the idea of the virtuous circle is the experience of anyone who has played a sport in a team, sung in a choir or pulled together with others to survive a crisis – common sense.

When we see people cooperating together in the virtuous circle, we can see that, individually and together, they display the following traits:

> The ability to *bear the other* (patient or colleague) *compassionately in mind.*

> The *imagination* to see how their actions or interventions might contribute to the well-being of the other.

> Confident belief in their own value and freedom to act.

> A repertoire of the right range of skills and knowledge to contribute.

All these things are seen when the nurse pauses to gently comb the patient's hair because he or she feels horrible, or when the nurse finds a way of reducing the embarrassment of incontinence for a proud patient or to calm the anxiety of a dementing old man who is frightened of a syringe. But all these things, and the virtuous circle, emerge in staff when the factors that can support or interfere with them are understood and managed, and when the psychological environment in which they work fosters the qualities discussed above.

The Challenge of Kindness

Kinship and kindness are what we are trying to cultivate, but everybody probably knows just how hard being 'family' in this way can be. The virtuous circle is vulnerable to breakdown – to 'failures of compassion', to coldness, neglect, even abuse – just as in Mid Staffordshire. To understand what makes compassion in healthcare difficult is not to arm staff with an excuse. What it may do is help everyone – from politicians, to management, to frontline staff – address these issues. For nurses, it may help them to preserve and protect compassion and to work with others to foster an environment that nourishes it.

To understand the challenge, we must start at the heart of healthcare work: with the nurse's encounter with illness and the wider state of illbeing in the patient. Nobody, from patients to their families, to neighbours or clinical staff, really *wants* to be with illness – with its often very unpleasant manifestations. Often, apart from the patient and her close persons, it is nurses who have to spend the most direct time with it. Pain, incontinence, wounds, bleeding, suppuration and smells, tumours, the signs of life slipping away – all of these things can prompt us to turn away, to feel anger, fear or disgust. Nurses have constantly to overcome such reactions, ensuring that their distaste or fear does not 'leak back' into the care they give, ensuring that, in overcoming the discomfort they feel, they do not shut themselves down emotionally or burn-out or become depressed. This self-overcoming (Tallis, 2005) is both an individual challenge and a *collective* one: so easily can the team or the group foster hardness, cynicism, disconnection from the patient or simply weary soul-lessness. That many people in healthcare, and perhaps society as a whole (when it is not calling nurses 'angels') underplay, or even deny, the hard emotional work involved in being with illness does not help.

Ill-being – the combination of physical, psychological and social dis-comfort the patient experiences – is much more complicated. Even a minor physical illness can arouse anger, depression and anxiety in a person. It can disturb relationships, interfere with the obligations and duties, and the pleasures, in their lives, provoking anxiety, anger, confusion or general loss of self-esteem. This disturbance can extend to involve those closest to the sick person. When nurses meet patients and their families, they encounter all this ill-being, often at times of high risk or suffering, when the anxiety and confusion are at their highest for everyone and where people manage these feelings in their own (not always obvious) ways.

Part of ill-being is *dependency* – something that many people have mixed feelings about: those who depend and those responsible for help-ing. Having to meet someone's needs (whether they are comfortable about depending on others or not) inevitably arouses anxiety in all of us – nurses included. Have we the time, emotional resources, the skill or the patience to meet these needs? What if we get it wrong? When that person is far from an open book, known only fleetingly, hard to 'read' in terms of what his or her sense and experience of and way of managing ill-being is like, then the challenge for the nurse in making a compassionate connection with the patient is great. Of course, the person in the bed or the treatment room may also be frightened or aggressive; he or she might be an asylum seeker, a criminal, a person suffering from HIV, a person with learning disabilities or a person of a very different culture, class or race from that of the nurse. Meeting them in their ill-being as 'kin' can be a very com-plex affair. Again, that systems and people underestimate this complica-tion works actively against helping people get through it to engage with patients. From the early days of training, it is important for nurses to be able, without self-pity or excuse, to bear in mind the difficulty and per-sonal cost involved in making and sustaining compassionate connections with patients. That way, they are constantly in touch with an absolutely vital truth: *compassionate care goes missing mainly because it's difficult to do, not because people are bad, lazy or stupid.*

The Needs of Staff

All of us are complicated people. We have the capacity to connect com-passionately and creatively with each other or to flee such connection, to fight, to become hardened. Neuroscience shows that we are built that way

(Gilbert, 2009). We all bring our needs, motives (not all of them generous), our blind spots and our ability to bear and face our feelings or to ignore and suppress them, to our work. This makes us all vulnerable to falling into bad habits: the staff in Mid Staffordshire Hospital were people like us. As individuals, we need, with the support of our colleagues and the systems around us, to manage the things that interfere with our capacity to engage together in the virtuous circle or worse, bring out the ungenerous, neglectful or even abusive sides of us.

Another perspective we need is to understand that the motivating power of kinship can work in two very different ways: it can prompt us to engage compassionately with others or to withdraw and exclude. When kinship emerged in the evolution towards modern human societies, it began as a relatively narrow and exclusive phenomenon: our fellow feeling, connection and cooperation extended only to our 'blood relatives', or the immediate family. Other families were beyond the boundaries of our sense of kinship; often competitors for scarce resources, even enemies. When we began, as hunters and gatherers or as pastoralist cultivators of crops, to cooperate beyond and between different blood families, we took a large step. On the one hand, we could readily see that our collective thriving depended on cooperating, but on the other we needed to develop ways of managing the tendency to pursue narrower, more selfish interests. Such extended kinship depended on agreements, on rules about fairness, on ways of regulating behaviour to prevent breakdowns in cooperation (Boehm, 2012). In modern healthcare, this challenge is all around us. Not only are we constantly called upon to include 'the stranger' in our kinship group, but effective and compassionate work – the virtuous circle – depends on the cooperation of various 'families', nursing, doctors, managers or ward, departments and service teams, which can turn inwards, narrowing their focus to self-interest, even to the extent of undermining each other. We need, *ethically* and psychologically, sophisticated attitudes, especially in leadership – not just systems and procedures – to help us resist the tendency for the virtuous circle to break down in such ways.

This kind of 'widened' kinship requires constant attention and active work to sustain it. When extended and multiple family groups of chimpanzees in Gombe, Tanzania, were studied by Jane Goodall and her team in the 1960s, the researchers found collective expressions of tenderness, playfulness, mutual support and sharing, problem solving and solidarity. This contrasted with the behaviour of other apes. The team were shocked, though, when this loving togetherness collapsed before their eyes into violence and pitiless murderousness. Michael Chance suggests that it was probably the introduction of *competition* for bananas placed by the researchers to entice the chimps to come closer that spurred this particular collapse: the chimps began to compete to get them, and at the same time neglected and finally left off their mutuality, their play, the everyday habits that sustained the extended family culture. Competitive behaviour rapidly became ruthless violence (Chance, 1988). We now know that chimps, like humans, despite having the capacity for more tender, collective kinship than many other apes, are often capable of horrific violence. The paradox is that the creative, open, mutually attentive and compassionate 'culture' is probably *more* vulnerable to collapse into neglect and abuse than rigid, cold and self-protective cultures; but the cooperative and nurturing virtuous circle is not much seen in the latter settings, where the focus is to fend off threat.

The lesson here is that we must pay very careful attention to ensuring we do not disturb, distract from or pervert the habits, activities and interactions that sustain creative kinship, by introducing the wrong kind of 'incentives' or 'preoccupations' into the system. Indeed, we must value and pay attention to fostering the small and large habits of cooperation, goodwill and mutuality upon which the virtuous circle depends, across the healthcare system. Staff who spend time together, get to know each other and even 'play' together are more likely to be able to sustain compassion in their collective work than people who simply come together to perform their duties in a detached, mechanical manner. At a time when resources – money, people and time – are so pressurised, it is easy to fall into the trap of thinking that valuing 'task efficiency' in isolation from the health of the social system in healthcare will produce the kind of compassionate and effective service and care that we want.

Social psychology has shed further light on the ways our behaviour in groups can be shaped for good or ill. Group pressure can not only lead us to conform but can actually skew the way we *perceive*. Solomon Asch demonstrated that a group can not just persuade a person to agree that a line drawn on paper is shorter or longer than it really is, but under sustained pressure, the person actually *sees* it as the length the group is conspiring to get him or her to see (Asch, 1951). Experiments led by Philip Zimbardo showed how *role pressure* led to extremes of behaviour. He simulated a prison, with students taking the roles of prisoners and guards, but was forced to stop the experiment prematurely because the 'guards' had become sadistic and bullying, and the students playing the prisoners were at risk of serious depression, even suicide; repeated simulations confirmed these findings (Haney, Bank and Zimbardo, 1973). Similarly, Stanley Milgram's notorious experiments showed how perfectly 'civilised' volunteer students were persuaded, by people whose *authority* they trusted, to administer what they thought were real, life-threatening electronic shocks to fellow students (Milgram, 1963).

These and other experiments demonstrate just how much attention we need to give to supporting the people in the system to retain their individuality, to creating a group culture that sustains positive kinship and to exercising leadership that is open, challengeable and sensitive to how the exercise of authority can stifle individual conscience, freedom to think and act, and concern for others. In a profession such as nursing, with its complex hierarchies, demarcations of responsibility and authority, and dependency on each other from moment to moment, getting all this right can be very challenging. It requires attention and recognition in the first instance in order that it can be taken further by all of us, at all levels and in all professions.

Managing Anxiety

How anxiety is managed at all levels is crucial. If the encounter with illness and ill-being evokes strong anxieties, how much more are they amplified by feeling overworked; by a lack of sufficient resources and time to complete work; by deadlines to meet or externally imposed performance targets to hit; and by people moving too fast to communicate all but the basics? And, of course, being professionals, nurses tend to get on with the work, overlooking the ways in which these anxieties are affecting them as people, often not noticing how their attention, patience, empathy – their capacity for kindness – are being diminished. When the same thing is happening to one degree or another across all professionals and at all levels of the hierarchy, then we have a system which becomes less supportive of the virtuous circle and more vulnerable to vicious circles dominated by the negative processes identified by the social psychologists whose work was summarised earlier. Unmanaged anxiety makes for a rich breeding ground for conformity, 'just following orders', following procedures mechanically but without kindness. Even worse, anxious people, unsupported, can become self-obsessed, distracted, angry and punitive. Anxiety will not just go away – though humane leadership, supportive relationships and well-organised, properly resourced services can help reduce and manage it. Even then, it is important that individual nurses be helped to develop the self-awareness to note how they are feeling and to think about how they are acting. Effective personal supervision, that integrates attention to tasks, skills and performance, with consideration of how individuals are managing themselves as people in their roles, is vital (Hawkins and Shohet, 2006). Training in various forms of *mindfulness*, especially Compassionate Mind training, which helps us look after ourselves and regulate our feelings, is also helpful (Gilbert, 2009). A range of small-group reflective approaches can also make a useful contribution.

Anxiety, though, also needs managing at the level of relationships – of teamwork, the way services interact and the way the organisation works. A team can become a place that helps its members manage their anxiety, be present and heard as individuals, think about patients as the complex people they are, plan how to work well together, and manage problems or failures in their work. At other times, the difficulty of the task can lead members to fall into passive dependency on individuals – sometimes the leader, sometimes not – to solve problems and reduce stress. Teams can descend into mistrust and conflict, with splits, alliances, withdrawal and spectatorism. Very commonly, teams can lapse into inertia – displacing the 'blame' for problems, and the power to resolve them, outside – to management or to other parts of the system. Most teams or groups move in and out of these states at some time – they are natural – but passively dependent people, people in conflict, people who blame or shift responsibility to others do not readily engage in the virtuous circle. Skills in managing oneself in the group and in leading groups to help them stay connected in active kinship are vital.

When anxiety is not managed situations such as that outlined below can result:

> An 80-year-old lady who has a few days before had a knee replacement lies in a bed in a hospital ward. In the corridor into the ward, stuck up on the wall, are a series of sheets of paper outlining a 'care pathway', with diagrams and procedures, about managing incontinence. This is what she and her visitors see as they pass in and out – not an explanation of knee treatment or rehabilitation and the roles of the multidisciplinary team, not the journey back to home and well-being. Above her bed is a slightly grubby and peeling sticker saying, 'Point of Care'. In fact, no one has spoken to her about after-care and recovery, about how physiotherapy and home care might work to help her recover. Often she has to wait uncomfortably to go to the toilet. She is told that she is blocking a bed and that they must find a way to move her on. How can this be?

Isobel Menzies-Lyth studied nursing in a London hospital and suggested that the way systems and procedures were organised had as much to do with managing anxiety as with quality of care, though people were unaware of this. But far from helping to build morale and making the task more manageable, many of the arrangements actually undermined these things: sickness levels and staff turnover were high. Unconscious attempts to cope with the anxiety in the task of caring for people led to ways of organising the work that broke the satisfying connection with patients, with their work and with each other (Menzies-Lyth, 1988). The example above shows this vividly – and suggests that we are also responding to anxiety that emerges not only from the difficult work of caring for the sick, but from scrutiny and criticism inside and outside the system. The incontinence pathway display (and all the time and work that had gone in to developing it) was almost certainly the product of worry in the hospital leadership generated by the Mid Staffordshire Report – which contained much about patients being left in soiled beds. The 'Point of Care' sticker probably expressed the need to assert proudly and publicly a commitment to 'seeing the person in the patient' – to assert it rather than to work out how to do it. And, no doubt, busy people spent lots of time spreading the word of the campaign – admirable as an intention, but having little connection with everyday work in this case.

Much of the life of a hospital or community healthcare team can be dominated by anxious distraction from patient care and the conversations and cooperation that make it possible. Much of the time, staff and those responsible for leading them are 'looking over their shoulders', away from the patients and each other. This might be to ensure that contract requirements and other national or local targets are met, that guidelines and procedures are being followed, that quality standards are high, and reported as such. At the very least, this preoccupation can lead to work that distracts from the patient – forms to fill, reports to produce, meetings to attend to monitor progress, and so on. But when people in the organisation, especially at the top, are anxious about financial performance, frightened of criticism, alarmed at the prospect of losing a contract or worried for their jobs, such distraction can become very dangerous indeed. Bullying behaviour, refusal to think about the realities of tight resources for staff and patients, and the consequences of systems and procedures introduced to improve efficiency, with a narrow focus on quantitative measures such as waiting times and discharge rates, can poison the emotional and social environment. The level of anxiety, combined with the narrow focus on particular issues, can lead to people treating each other as a means to an end, to manipulating facts to placate mistrustful seniors or outside scrutiny such as regulators, to turning a blind eye to unwanted or unforeseen consequences. Such a culture prevents staff from building and sustaining the virtuous circle.

The Patient Experience

It is not just staff who are affected by such a culture. In a system focused on procedures and guidelines for treating specific conditions, with timescales for 'throughput', efficiency and so on, many groups of patients find it more and more difficult to find their place as 'kin' in the system. Older people with multiple health problems; people with communication, learning or mental health difficulties; and people with complex needs rather than single conditions do not readily find the recognition and response they need as people in such a system. At the 'front line', nurses can then be caught in an almost unbearable tension between their sense of what their patients need and the pressure to ignore it.

It is crucial then for leaders – at all levels, from chief executive to 'shift senior' – to ensure that their anxiety does not lead to such a climate and that the unavoidable need to meet standards and performance targets, to satisfy regulatory requirements and to improve efficiency is never at the expense of the health of the relational system. This requires personal qualities of self-awareness and, above all, openness and honesty between colleagues – seniors, peers and juniors. Everyone needs to collaborate in keeping reality in mind.

Something that can help enormously is taking the time to 'hear the full story'. Our preoccupation with snapshot 'satisfaction surveys' – for patients or staff – with over-simplified measures such as the (quite sensible) 'friends and family test' can mean we lose touch with what we can do to strengthen the virtuous circle, to improve the quality and effectiveness of care. Hearing a patient's narrative – from the beginning of his or her illness through the whole process of receiving care – as a human story about the patient's experience, including, but not only, of care and treatment – engages our imagination, empathy and problem-solving skills. Hearing staff stories – not just how they rate their organisation, but what their work is like for them – can draw together colleagues in shared understanding, in positive relationships, and, again, inspire constructive problem-solving and service improvement. This approach is central to the use of Schwartz Rounds, where staff share and reflect on their stories (Goodrich and Cornwell, 2008) (see Chapter 7).

Conclusion

Nurses have a hard task that can be immensely satisfying but which is fraught with difficult feelings, pressures and distractions. To work with the 'intelligent kindness' this chapter has been exploring, they need to do the following:

> Remember at all times that the quality of their work – and their morale – depends on the quality of their relationships with patients and colleagues as kin.

> Develop the habits of self-awareness and reflective practice that can help them manage themselves in their roles and relationships.

> Understand what happens in and between teams and groups, and develop an awareness of how they experience and operate in group settings.

> Have the courage to share their experience and perceptions.

And, above all, recognise leadership that understands that the quality, effectiveness and efficiency of services depends on the quality of relationships – between staff and patients and among staff – and has the commitment and skill to lead accordingly.

References

Asch, S. E. (1951) 'Effects of Group Pressure upon the Modification and Distortion of Judgement', in H. Guetzkow (ed.) *Groups, Leadership and Men* (Pittsburgh: Carnegie Press).

Ballatt, J. and P. Campling (2011) *Intelligent Kindness: Reforming the Culture of Healthcare* (London: Royal College of Psychiatrists).

Boehm, C. (2012) *Moral Origins: The Evolution of Virtue, Altruism and Shame* (New York: Basic Books).

Bowlby, J. (1999/1969) *Attachment. Attachment and Loss*, Vol. 1, 2nd edn (New York: Basic Books).

Chance, M.R.A. (1988) *Social Fabrics of the Mind* (London: Lawrence Erlbaum).

Cole-King, A. and K. G. Harding (2001) 'Psychological Factors and Delayed Healing in Chronic Wounds', *Psychosomatic Medicine*, 63: 216–20.

Cooper, M. (2008) *Essential Research Findings in Counselling and Psychotherapy* (London: Sage).

Department of Health (DH) (2012a) *Compassion in Practice: Nursing, Midwifery and Care Staff, Our Vision and Strategy* (London: HMSO).

Department of Health (DH) (2012b) *Transforming Care: A National Response to Winterbourne View Care Home* (London: HMSO).

Francis, R. (2010) *Independent Inquiry into Care Provided by Mid Staffordshire NHS Foundation Trust, January 2005–March 2009* (London: HMSO).

Francis, R. (2013) *Report of the Mid Staffordshire NHS Foundation Trust Public Inquiry* (London: The Stationery Office).

Gilbert, P. (2009) *The Compassionate Mind: A New Approach to Life's Challenges* (London: Constable and Robinson).

Goodrich, J. and J. Cornwell (2008) *Seeing the Person in the Patient*, The Point of Care Review Paper (London: King's Fund).

Haney, C., W. C. Bank and P. G. Zimbardo (1973) 'Interpersonal Dynamics in a Simulated Prison', *International Journal of Criminology and Penology*, 1: 69–97.

Hawkins, P. and R. Shohet (2006) *Supervision in the Helping Professions* (Maidenhead: Open University Press).

Holmes, J. (1993) *John Bowlby and Attachment Theory* (London and New York: Routledge).

Menzies-Lyth, I. (1988) 'The Functions of Social Systems as a Defence Against Anxiety: A Report on a Study of the Nursing Service of a General Hospital', *Human Relations*, 1959(13): 95–121; reprinted in *Containing Anxiety in Institutions: Selected Essays, Vol. 1* (London: Free Association Books).

Milgram, S. (1963) 'Behavioural Study of Obedience', *Journal of Abnormal and Social Psychology*, 67: 371–78.

NHS England 2014 Winterbourne View – Time for Change. Transforming the commissioning of services for people with learning disabilities and/or autism. NHS England, London. www.england.nhs.uk/wp-content/uploads/2014/11/transforming-commissioning-services.pdf, accessed 16 March 2016).

patientopinion.org.uk, last accessed 20 December 2014.

Rendelmeir, D. A., J. Molin and R. J. Tibshirani (1995) 'A Randomised Trial of Compassionate Care for the Homeless in an Emergency Department', *Lancet*, 345: 1131–4.

Tallis, R. (2005) *Hippocratic Oaths: Medicine and Its Discontents* (London: Atlantic Books).

Weinman, J., M. Ebrecht, S. Scott, J. Walburn and J. Dyson (2008) 'Enhanced Wound Healing after Emotional Disclosure Intervention', *British Journal of Health Psychology*, 13(1): 95–102.

6

The Components of Compassion

Marjorie Ghisoni (Formerly Lloyd)

Introduction

This chapter shares some of the findings from a recent PhD study which investigated the involvement of mental health service users and their carers in practice. In this chapter, the discussion of what constitutes compassion in practice is extended to explore some of the components of compassionate nursing care. However, the theoretical, theological and philosophical roots of compassion are not discussed as they have already been addressed in Chapters 2 and 3. In this chapter, social research which used a narrative methodology to identify the actions of compassionate practice is described as a way of measuring compassion. The aim of the qualitative study was to capture the everyday experiences of long-term mental health service users and their carers. However, because the study was about service user involvement, the findings can be applied in other fields of nursing practice.

The study focused on discovering what service users needed to become more involved in their own care. Three areas of practice were identified where compassion towards others could be demonstrated. These were a *universal* understanding of each other's strengths and goals, a recognition of the *diversity* that we all share as individuals and in groups and a collaborative approach towards hope of *recovery* in mental health skills and abilities. Each of these areas was drawn out of the study as being an important theme when involving people in care. Each can also be a way of demonstrating compassionate care and how we approach people as professionals and as individual human beings in helping them regain some control over their lives. In mental health services, compassionate care is also a way of demonstrating recovery-focused practices as recommended in many national and local policy guidelines. Recovery-focused practices in mental healthcare centre on outcomes which differ from those for people with physical health problems who might expect to be cured of their illness. In mental health, the focus of recovery is on ensuring that people with mental illness retain a sense of hope and optimism so that they can live with and gain control over the debilitating symptoms associated with severe and enduring mental illness (DH, 2004, 2006). The mental health practitioner and author Watkins (2009) identifies how compassionate care might appear in practice. He recommends a humanistic, psychological approach to compassionate practice in mental health:

> What sustains the human spirit through such troubled states of mind, when distress is so enveloping that everyday living becomes difficult, if not impossible, is the empathic and compassionate presence of another who can be a caretaker of hope. (p. ix)

The literal meaning of compassion is to share (*com*-panion) the thoughts and feelings (*passion*) that another person is expressing at any given time, and nurses in all areas of practice need to demonstrate this to the best of their ability. In the findings of the Francis Report (2013), the recognition of a lack of compassion that can result from burnout or compassion fatigue is discussed as a barrier to good-quality care and a major risk to the safety of staff and the people in their care. The Francis Report (2013) makes many recommendations (see Chapter 1); however, one issue repeatedly referred to is putting the patient first.

> The overarching value and principle of the NHS Constitution should be that patients are put first, and everything done by the NHS and everyone associated with it should be informed by this ethos. (p. 67)

In what follows, the way this can be approached in mental health services is examined.

Service User Involvement in Mental Health Services

Involving service users in the design of mental health services has been a key concern of organisational and empirical activity focused on developing better-quality services. A major policy driver of this approach to person-centred and recovery-orientated services was *The Ten Essential Capabilities A Framework for the Whole of the Mental Health Workforce* (DH, 2004), which was developed as a guide for nurses and other mental health practitioners to help them take a more compassionate approach in mental healthcare. The Department of Health (DH) (2004: 1) identified that

> [t]he shift in culture in services towards choice, person-centredness, and mental health promotion is a key imperative. People who use services and their

families continue to report not being listened to, being marginal to assessment and care planning and being rendered helpless rather than helped by the service.

In addition to this change in policy, there were growing concerns about community care for the mentally ill, the use of mental health law to detain people against their will and the lack of evidence-based treatments in different parts of the UK and elsewhere in the world (DH, 1998, 2006, 2007). At the time these major policy changes were taking place in the UK, the World Health Organization (WHO, 2008) predicted that by 2030 depression would be the leading cause of ill health, resulting in more people taking sick leave from work because of mental health problems than for any other major disease. The growing burden of mental illness on society has therefore increased the need for a compassionate approach to mental healthcare which can be measured using recovery outcomes. Such outcomes should reflect that people who suffer from mental health problems need to be involved in their care in order to help them to recover and live meaningful lives (Lloyd and Carson, 2012).

Involving service users in the design and delivery of care should, in theory, prevent people who use mental health services being *rendered helpless* by the very service that they most need help from to regain control of their lives. Mental health nurses, and the nursing profession more widely, must also take responsibility and become accountable for always acting in the best interest of the people they care for and supporting them in the healing process (Nursing and Midwifery Council [NMC], 2008). In order to do this in practice, the boundaries between patient and nurse become obscured by the needs of both. For example, Gadow (1996: 8) asserts:

> Nurses perhaps more than other professionals recognise the illusion of the private public distinction. In clinical situations where personal needs are attended by strangers, where patient vulnerability and professional objectivity collide and coexist the ordinary boundary between public and private disappears.

When the boundaries in practice are blurred, the nurse and the patient become involved in each other's stories as they develop the therapeutic relationship and identify shared goals. Such an intimate relationship is recognised by some nurse theorists as unique and essential to effective nursing practice (Gadow, 1996; Holloway and Freshwater, 2007). As the nurse and the patient share their stories, they develop a narrative that is based on the knowledge and expertise of both (Mishler, 1986). In order to incorporate this shared approach in practice, a narrative design was used that was essentially about listening to service users' stories (Frank,

1997; Riesmann, 2008) and considering how these might contribute towards genuine involvement practice. This is discussed further later in the chapter, to illustrate how nurses can involve people more in their care by developing a compassionate approach in practice. Clark, Glasby and Lester (2004) identify the benefits of service user involvement as the social capital of working with others, recovering skills that have been lost and developing new skills and hence the chance to earn a living. They also identified an improvement in self-confidence and an opportunity to reflect upon skills gained. Involving service users in their own care and in teaching and research also demonstrates a willingness to listen and a commitment to emancipatory and empowering practice. Research on service user involvement was carried out prior to this study which provided background information for the work. (For more information, see Lloyd and Carson [2005, 2012] and Lloyd [2006, 2007].) Gathering patient stories, however, is just the beginning of the process of genuine and compassionate service user involvement. Such stories can then build into a narrative of involvement practice that continues to grow from recognising the resonance and rapport between and within personal and professional relationships. Such resonance is an important part of narrative research (Frank, 1997; Gadow, 1996; Riessman, 2008).

Narrative Theory and Research

Narrative theory, like compassion, is not a new concept and has a history as long as people have been able to write, as it became a natural process of recording history and experiences (Frank, 1997; Riessman, 2008). The use of narratives in research and practice in healthcare, however, has been criticised for not being objective or scientifically based (Holloway and Freshwater, 2007). In reality and in practice, Holloway and Freshwater (2007) suggest that nurses and other professionals increasingly find research from the clinical fields hard to translate into everyday encounters with people who are often vulnerable and confused. Narrative research may be useful in addressing this area of practice, as both researcher and participant co-create the data, empowering both in the process (Mishler, 1986; Frank, 1997; Riessman, 2008). Subjective ideas that are developed from individual stories can then be translated into objective outcomes that can be measured in practice.

When carrying out narrative research, the researcher and the participants both become part of the findings that are woven together during analysis with existing evidence, theory and policy (Holloway and Freshwater, 2007; Riessman, 2008). This approach may therefore help nurses apply theory to practise in a more comfortable and compassionate way, identifying and addressing the needs of both service users and staff. For the participants in this study, the co-creation approach helped them to articulate and explore what really mattered to them, if they were to become more involved in mental health nursing practice.

Narrative approaches to both research and practice have been used in psychology and counselling (Mishler, 1986) as well as medicine (Hurwitz, Greenhalgh and Skultans, 2004). Narrative medicine is a growing discipline which involves listening to people's stories and experiences to give meaning to their suffering (Hurwitz et al., 2004). However, in the busy clinical environment the individual stories of people are not always heard, may be ignored and even actively suppressed (Kleinman, 1988; Church, 1995). This prevents nurses and other healthcare staff providing compassionate care. For example when reflecting on a clinical team meeting that he had been involved in, Kleinman noted:

> There were ghosts present in the room. I am sure of it. For each case discussed, the shadows of the players in the family tragedies and comedies and the melodramas in the workplace seemed to float in the corners of the room, unseen and unheard. (Kleinman, 1988: 175)

Such unseen and unheard narratives were the focus of this study, which has similarities to the work of Church (1995), who examined *Forbidden Narratives* in her research on service user involvement in mental health services in Canada. This autobiographical account explored the sometimes uncomfortable areas of researching our own practice and developing an honest and trustworthy approach to gathering data. Church (1995) discovered that it was the things that were not said, as Kleinman (1988) observed, that were perhaps the most important. Church described these important but often unnoticed sections of data as the *white spaces* between the text of the recorded data which warranted further interpretation. Using a narrative approach to the data-gathering process, the white spaces become filled with interpretation and analysis in order to create a *critical conversation* as a methodology for both research and practice (Lloyd and Carson, 2012).

In developing a narrative approach for this study, it was important to ensure that service user voices were heard and their accounts informed the findings. Moreover it was important to involve participants who had a story to tell from their years of experience in and out of mental health services. Such experience generates a wealth of information because, as Riessman (2008) suggests, 'It is generally acknowledged in the human sciences that the researcher does not find narratives but participates in their creation' (p. 2).

This is an empowering process for both the researcher and the participant (Mishler, 1986). Listening to people, with sympathy and empathy, creates a compassionate dialogue that is perhaps absent in other forms of research (Nussbaum, 2001).

Consequently, third-sector groups were approached to take part in the study in which a rich variety of data were gathered. This was collected in group interviews in an effort to ensure that a conversation took place that examined current services and could also be analysed at a later date. This narrative approach led to the development of what was eventually termed Critical Conversations (Lloyd and Carson, 2012) as a methodology for narrative research which could also be used in everyday practice. This approach is also useful for researchers interested in discovering more about how compassion can be demonstrated in practice. Empowering nurses and service users to create a dialogue about their practice by weaving together individual stories enables us to make visible the components of compassionate nursing care (see Figure 6.1).

Methodological Design

The research was designed to capture the experiences of people who were already familiar with the mental health system, to discover how they could become more involved in their own care. Participation and personalisation are major drivers in current psychiatric care, intended to shift the focus from the service to the person (DH, 2004, 2006; Lloyd, 2012). Personalisation is an attempt to drive services towards a more compassionate approach in identifying and understanding what individual people need to recover their mental health. To do this, we need to know about their experiences in relation to empowering practice. We are perhaps not as aware as we should be as nurses of the everyday assumptions that we make about people in our care. Developing compassionate practice requires us to explore our assumptions and to develop a reflective analytical approach to our everyday conversations with people. The narrative approach outlined earlier enables all participants to develop a critical conversation that can uncover what might have otherwise been left in the white spaces of such assumptions (Church, 1995; Frank, 1997; Watkins, 2009).

The sample of people who participated in the study was purposive in that all had many years' experience of mental health services and a diagnosis of a serious mental illness which meant they had become disabled by their illness. They had all been known to services for some time. Participants were invited to take part in a group interview in a place that was familiar to them so that they would feel more able to discuss their experiences openly. In developing a narrative approach, Holloway and Freshwater (2007) and Riessman (2008) suggest that semi-structured group interviews can be used to enable people to tell their own personal stories. These initial data were then subject to thematic analysis to identify involvement practices as components of compassion that can be observed and consequently measured in nursing practice (see Figure 6.1).

The analysis of the data was conducted during and after the interviews took place as the researcher and participants co-created the data (Mishler, 1986). The data were gathered by tape-recording the interviews, which were later transcribed verbatim and reread by the principal researcher to discover codes and themes. Riessman (2008) argues that thematic analysis is a useful method for sorting through the vast amount of data to find common occurrences. Once identified, these codes and themes were analysed further through a deconstructive process and then reconstructed into a shared narrative of service users' experiences of involvement in mental health practice (Holloway and Freshwater, 2007; Lloyd and Carson, 2012).

The study considered the ethical implications as the participants in this study were all vulnerable people who suffered with, or supported someone suffering from, a serious mental illness over many years. It was important when asking vulnerable people to take part in research that they understood what they were being asked to do and that it was unlikely they would come to any harm by participating (Riessman, 2008).

The Findings

The following themes were identified during the transcription and analysis of the data until data saturation was reached and no new codes emerged (Guba and Lincoln, 1994). In qualitative research, this method of analysis is common in helping the researcher get as close as possible to the data while generating a new narrative from the findings. The themes of universality, diversity and recovery were created during analysis and in order to group the data into areas of practice that were visible to both the nurse and the service users. Narrative research explores what is hidden in the accounts of service users and exposes areas of practice that could involve more compassion being shown towards the needs of service users (Church, 1995; Frank, 1997; Watkins, 2009). The three themes are now discussed in more detail.

Universality as Collaborative Practice

Patient involvement in healthcare is not a new idea and can be found in both policy and theoretical guidelines. For example in nurse education, the professional regulator, the NMC requires all education providers to demonstrate service user involvement in programme development and the education of nursing students.

The DH (1998, 2004, 2006) has also consistently suggested that mental health service users should be fully involved in their care and that nurses, as their care coordinators, should be able to identify and share goals through interaction with service providers and service users. This universal approach is then shared across local health and social care providers to improve communication and to develop services that best meet the needs of local service users. In this study, service users and carers identified stability within relationships as being very important for their involvement. In the following extract, a service user explains how important it is to know that there is someone who understands the need for stability and continuity in the nurse–patient relationship: 'It's just knowing that there's that stability behind everything, that you are there, whatever' (P1G2).

In mental health services, stability is made visible or objective as a universal need for both service users and service providers, when, for much of the time, care may appear to be in chaos. Nurses who provide stability by being available and in regular contact with service users demonstrate universal compassion as a sympathetic understanding of service users' needs (Nussbaum, 2001; Watkins, 2009). A stable relationship also provides the opportunity to get to know a person, and in nursing, Gadow (1996) suggests, the personal and professional boundaries may become blurred in an attempt to understand the diverse needs of the individual. The next theme explores the component of diversity within compassionate practice and indicates that if diversity is not recognised then discrimination may become more evident in practice.

Diversity or Discrimination

Most healthcare professionals understand that people are individual human beings with their own beliefs and morals that influence how they live their lives (Holloway and Freshwater, 2007; Watkins, 2009). As well as identifying universal needs, this study also found that service users wanted to be treated as individuals and not assumed to have the same needs as everyone else. When diverse needs are ignored, services can become too medicalised and clinical in treating everyone the same (Kleinman, 1988; Church, 1995; Clark et al., 2004; Hurwitz et al., 2004).

Nussbaum (2001) and Watkins (2009) suggest that compassion can be demonstrated by developing an empathetic understanding of the diverse needs of people in a genuine attempt to encourage recovery and prevent categorisation and consequent discrimination. The following participant suggested that diversity should be seen as a strength in the relationship between nurses and service users and not used to discriminate between them.

> But discrimination has got nothing to do with it, it's not because we have mental health problems it's because these are staff and we are not staff, we don't work in your environment, we have no experience of your environment other than using it and therefore we need training in a different way, and that's common sense it is not discrimination is it? (P1G1)

This service user was trying to explain how diversity can become a barrier (or white space) if not recognised. Service users and nurses have different needs and different beliefs and ways of working. This is to be expected if we are serious about diversity in healthcare practice. It is not about treating everyone the same, but about recognising different needs. Nurses can demonstrate compassionate care by recognising individual needs and finding ways to support the service user in addressing them (Clark et al., 2004; Hurwitz et al., 2004; Watkins, 2009). Identifying the diverse needs and strengths of a person also demonstrates a compassionate approach towards individual recovery, as the next theme illustrates.

Recovery or Rehabilitation?

For many years, in healthcare we have sought to rehabilitate people in order to help them regain their lives and independence to varying degrees (DH, 2004, 2006). The focus on rehabilitation, however, can be more a controlling than a collaborative approach, where the professional tells people what they need to do to recover (Holloway and Freshwater, 2007; Barker, 2009). Rehabilitation in this sense can be quite disempowering for individuals who may be afraid to make any decisions about their own health needs without consulting a professional first. Mental healthcare and discrimination, when discussed in this way, become a moral responsibility of the nurse. This responsibility can be the difference between whether a person recovers or not (Clark et al., 2004; Watkins, 2009). Compassionate mental health nursing can be demonstrated by exploring the diverse needs of individuals and how their needs can be addressed in order to help them recover their independence. In the study, one service user reflected upon his recovery:

> I remember my brother coming to see me at a time when I was having these awful side effects, and he said it was awful to see but I see it as, how can I put it, I don't regret being ill I see it as part of me, you know it is who I am. (Peter, ex-service user)

In this extract, Peter wants to be accepted and to accept himself for who he is now, and that is what recovery means to him. In mental healthcare, recovery does not mean *cure* but *care* that is diverse and compassionate in meeting individual needs (DH, 2004, 2006). Mental healthcare can, however, still instil fear in people, which prevents them from discussing their individual needs with other people and professionals, thus hindering their own recovery (Barker, 2009; Watkins, 2009).

Preventing people from recovering may appear to be an odd idea to acknowledge in contemporary mental health services. Nevertheless, if the environment in which nurses are working prevents them from practising in a recovery-orientated way, they can quickly begin to suffer from compassion fatigue or burnout, which prevents nurses from developing a compassionate approach to their care (Holloway and Freshwater, 2007; Austin et al., 2009; Barker, 2009; Watkins, 2009; DH, 2013).

Compassion Fatigue

Austin et al. (2009) suggest that compassion fatigue occurs when persons working with people who have been or are severely distressed, for whatever reason, become overwhelmed by the raw emotions and feelings of others. As a protective measure, they then begin to distance themselves from people who are stressed or very demanding. Compassion fatigue can be observed in the behaviour of the people affected who may display the following behaviours: they might be short-tempered, irritable, critical, judgemental, tired, agitated, neglectful of personal care and hygiene, careless with their work and money, and lack appetite, drink more alcohol and smoke more, spend more time sleeping and enjoy life less (Douglas, 2010). Although similar to some of the symptoms of depression, compassion fatigue should not be treated with medication in the first instance but in the reorganisation of the working environment (DH, 2013). Staff should be encouraged to take regular breaks and time out from practice and should be treated in a compassionate way by their managers (Austin et al., 2009). If self-compassion does not occur, then safety on the ward is jeopardised, and the quality of practice declines regardless of how many staff are available (Douglas, 2010; DH, 2013). In order to develop a compassionate working environment, the same three areas of practice described above could be used to measure the compassion shown towards staff so that they can in turn be more compassionate towards the people in their care (Nussbaum, 2001; Holloway and Freshwater, 2007; Watkins, 2009).

The three areas of involvement practices identified above make visible the components of compassion in nursing care. In recognising the diverse needs of staff and working in collaboration towards shared or universal goals for the service environment, we can enable nursing staff to recover their hope and courage to do a good job (Austin et al., 2009). In developing compassionate environments, managers and service providers can provide evidence for the compassionate care of service users (Douglas, 2010). In developing compassionate practice therefore, it is important to be able to recognise compassion fatigue in oneself and in others so that it can be addressed before it becomes too damaging (DH, 2013).

The components of compassionate practice can all be demonstrated in nursing practice and observed in everyday life (see Figure 6.1). Nussbaum (2001) suggests compassion consists of empathy, sympathy and knowledge, which can also be objectively measured. Nussbaum (2001) has since developed a capabilities approach as an ethical tool for measuring compassion by identifying basic human rights that belong to every one of us. For this study, the following components were created from the analysis of the data.

Components of Compassionate Nursing Care

Universality

Exploring collaborative ways to identify shared goals and expectations

Diversity

Identifying individual strengths and needs to facilitate coping and avoid discrimination

Recovery

Providing hope for recovery and role-modelling self-compassion

---

Figure 6.1 Components of Compassionate Nursing Care.

Conclusion

The study reported in this chapter was carried out during turbulent times in the National Health Service (NHS), and so allowances must be made for the stress that both staff and service users were under in adapting to such change. For its part, the government also recognises that the last thing people need now is more change (DH, 2013), but service provision and delivery must become more focused on the needs of service users if we are to demonstrate compassionate nursing care. This can be achieved by developing a critical stance towards current practice and having everyday conversations about compassionate care. Developing such critical conversations will help nurses to identity and measure compassionate practice that recognises the needs of both the nurse and the service user in planning care that respects diverse needs and individual recovery. People can only be the best that they can be at any given time, and this includes professional staff. Compassionate practice does, however, need to be supported and measured in the working environment. In order to develop compassionate practice, all nurses must be able to make visible the invisible and recognise the components of compassionate practice, outlined above, in their everyday practice.

References

Austin, W., E. Goble, B. Leier and P. Byrne (2009) 'Compassion Fatigue: The Experience of Nurses', *Ethics and Social Welfare* 3(2): 195–214.

Barker, P. (2009) 'The Politics of Caring', in P. Barker (ed.) *Psychiatric and Mental Health Nursing: The Craft of Caring* (London: Hodder Arnold) Chapter 84.

Church, K. (1995) *Forbidden Narratives Critical Autobiography as Social Science* (London: Routledge).

Clark, M., J. Glasby and H. Lester (2004) 'Cases for Change User Involvement in Mental Health Services and Research', *Research Policy & Planning*, 22(2): 31–8.

Department of Health (DH) (1998) *Modernising Mental Health Services: Safe, Sound and Supportive* (London: HMSO).

Department of Health (DH) (2004) *The Ten Essential Shared Capabilities* (London: HMSO).

Department of Health (DH) (2006) *From Values to Action. The Chief Nursing Officer's Review of Mental Health Nursing* (London: HMSO).

Department of Health (DH) (2008) *Refocusing the Care Programme Approach* (London: The Stationery Office).

Department of Health (DH) (2013) *Report of the Mid Staffordshire NHS Foundation Trust. Public Inquiry.* Executive summary, R. Francis [QC] (London: The Stationery Office).

Douglas, K. (2010) 'When Caring Stops, Staffing Doesn't Really Matter', *Nurse Economics*, 28(6): 415–19.

Frank, A. (1997) *The Wounded Storyteller: Body Illness and Ethics* (Chicago University Press).

Francis, R. (2013) *Report of the Mid Staffordshire NHS Foundation Trust Public Inquiry* (London: The Stationery Office).

Gadow, S. (1996) 'Ethical Narratives in Practice', *Nursing Science Quarterly*, 9(8): 8–9.

Guba, E. G. and Y. S. Lincoln (1994) 'Competing Paradigms in Qualitative Research', in N. K. Denzin and Y. S. Lincoln (eds) *Handbook of Qualitative Research* (London: Sage), chapter 6, pp. 105–17.

Holloway, I. and D. Freshwater (2007) *Narrative Research in Nursing* (Oxford: Blackwell).

Hurwitz, B., T. Greenhalgh and V. Skultans (2004) *Narrative Research in Health and Illness* (Oxford: Blackwell).

Kleinman, A. (1988) *The Illness Narratives: Suffering, Healing and the Human Condition* (New York: USA Basic Books).

Lloyd, M. (2006) 'Involving Service Users in Research', unpublished Fellowship Report (Cardiff: Health Professions Wales).

Lloyd, M. (2007) 'Empowerment in the Interpersonal Field: Discourses of Acute Mental Health Nurses', *Journal of Psychiatric and Mental Health Nursing*, 14: 485–94.

Lloyd, M. (2012) *Practical Care Planning for Personalised Mental Health Care* (Maidenhead: Open University Press).

Lloyd, M. and A. Carson (2005) 'Culture Shift: Carer Empowerment and Cooperative Enquiry', *Journal of Psychiatric and Mental Health Nursing*, 12(2): 187–91.

Lloyd, M. and A. Carson (2012) 'Critical Conversations: Developing a Methodology for Service User Involvement in Mental Health Nursing', *Nurse Education Today*, 32(2): 151–5.

Mishler, E. G. (1986) *Research Interviewing: Context and Narrative* (London: Harvard University Press).

Nussbaum, M. (2001) *Upheavals of Thought. The Intelligence of Emotions* (Cambridge: Cambridge University Press).

Riessman, C. K. (2008) *Narrative Methods for the Human Sciences* (London: Sage).

Watkins, P. (2009) *Mental Health Practice A Guide to Compassionate Care*, 2nd edn (London: Elsevier).

World Health Organization (WHO) (2008) The Global Burden of Disease 2004 Update. Geneva.

7

Improving Patients' Experience: The Point of Care 2007–14

Jocelyn Cornwell

Introduction

A much-quoted, accessible definition of *compassion* is 'a deep awareness of the suffering of another coupled with the wish to relieve it' (Chochinov, 2007: 186). In this way, people can express compassion towards others when they demonstrate an understanding of their suffering, by being there with them in some way that makes their pain more bearable (Firth-Cozens and Cornwell, 2009). Conventionally considered an attribute of individuals, we can also think of compassion as the ethos of a team or the defining quality of a service.

We can identify three distinctive sources of suffering when people are injured or ill (Mylod and Lee, 2013):

1. *Unavoidable* suffering associated with the diagnosis, which includes the symptoms of the disease, loss of functioning and the fear and anxiety connected to receiving the diagnosis itself.

2. *Unavoidable* suffering associated with treatment, which may include, for example, post-operative pain, loss of functioning and the fear and anxiety associated with the unavoidable disruption to normal life.

3. *Avoidable* suffering associated with dysfunctional aspects of the health-care delivery system. This may include, for example, misdiagnosis; delays in diagnosis; iatrogenic harm; intended or unintended indifference to the patient; infringements of the patient's privacy and dignity; the experience of avoidable pain, fear and anxiety; and unnecessary delay and waits.

Following these definitions, we can define a compassionate health-care service as one where the physical environment, the organisation of care and the behaviour of staff are intentionally designed to reduce the avoidable suffering and distress associated with the dysfunctional aspects of the healthcare delivery system.

The Point of Care Foundation sees compassion as both an attribute of individuals and a defining quality of a service. Listed here are the questions we want to answer:

1. Is it possible intentionally to design compassionate awareness and relief of the suffering of others into healthcare delivery?

2. And if so, is it possible to sustain the awareness of the suffering of others and the desire to relieve it in large numbers of staff over the long term?

In the first phase of work, the Point of Care was a programme of research and action at the King's Fund, the London-based think tank (2007–13). In 2013, it separated from the King's Fund to become the Point of Care Foundation, an independent charity that has the vision of radical improvement in the way we care and are cared for as patients, to create a truly human-centred approach.

When we began in 2007, the context for our work in the NHS and other health systems was different. At the end of the twentieth century, albeit belatedly, healthcare systems in high-income economies woke up to the risks associated with medical treatment and were looking to other high-risk industries for insights into the science of human error and to learn how to measure and reduce so-called 'patient safety incidents'. The Institute of Medicine's seminal report *To Err is Human* (1999) stimulated a global patient safety movement and opened the doors to research into patient safety problems and the development of practical tools for monitoring safety incidents and reducing harm.

However, in the early years of this century, patients' experience of care attracted comparatively little attention. In the United States, organisations such as the Picker Institute and the Planetree Association campaigned for patient-centred care. In the UK – apart from the national patient survey programme and the work carried out in nursing development units (Redfern et al., 1997) – not a lot was happening. When we started at the King's Fund, our own advisors warned that 'patient-centred care' was an attractive idea, but our efforts to focus attention on patients' experience of care were unlikely to succeed because it was not a priority for policymakers or NHS senior leaders.

Since then, the landscape has altered radically: patients' experience of care is now a policy and management priority. In 2008, the Darzi Report defined quality healthcare as care that is safe, clinically excellent and '*personalised*' (meaning tailored to the individual patient), and reframed the goal of the NHS as being to improve quality (DH, 2008). Following that report, there have been a number of further developments:

- ➤ Investment in research into patients' experience of care, with significant studies of the experiences of people in vulnerable groups, NHS organisational cultures, and the roles and experience of healthcare assistants.

- ➤ Papers published on staff experience (Boorman, 2009), staff and patient experience (Goodrich and Cornwell, 2008) and compassionate care (Firth-Cozens and Cornwell, 2009; Adamson et al., 2012).

- ➤ The development of innovative methods for capturing patients' feedback on their care experiences and a burgeoning market for providers of patient feedback services (Patient Opinion and I Want Great Care, for example).

- ➤ A national debate about the best and most cost-effective methods of measuring patients' experience and using patients' experience data to drive change (Coulter, Fitzpatrick and Cornwell, 2009; Dr Foster Ltd., 2010; Robert and Cornwell, 2011).

- ➤ The development and evaluation of patient-focused quality-improvement methods (Bate and Robert, 2007; Locock et al., 2014; King's Fund, 2014; NHS Institute Worldwide, 2014).

This chapter reflects on the work of the Point of Care Foundation. Section 1 discusses the intellectual foundations, theoretical perspectives, concepts and definitions that underpin our work, and the way we framed the problems we wish to solve. Section 2 presents our practical work with NHS organisations and front-line staff, and the lessons we have learned about what helps and what hinders improvement. The concluding section reflects on the future for efforts to advance compassionate care.

Intellectual Foundations: Language, Concepts and Definitions

At the outset, the Point of Care Programme adopted the Institute of Medicine's definition of patient experience (Institute of Medicine, 2001), because it was based on research with patients and their families (Delbanco, 1996). The Institute of Medicine defined patient experience as one dimension of healthcare quality, a complex, multidimensional phenomenon in its own right (the others being timeliness, equity, clinical quality, safety, access and efficiency), made up of these elements:

1. Respect for individual preferences

2. Emotional support

3. Involvement of family and friends

4. Physical comfort

5. Education training and communication

6. Information

7. Coordination and transitions of care.

The National Quality Board/Department of Health patient experience framework for England (2011) is based on the same dimensions but lists them in a different order and includes *access* to services. The Department of Health (DH) framework comprises:

1. Respect for patient-centred values, preferences and expressed needs

2. Coordination and integration of care

3. Information, communication and education

4. Physical comfort

5. Emotional support

6. The involvement of family and friends

7. Transition and continuity

8. Access to care.

It is useful to note that in both frameworks patients' experience is made up of elements that are *relational* (i.e. they are about *how* care is delivered) and elements that are *transactional* (they are about *what* is delivered). For the Point of Care, and for this volume, it is worth noting that compassion is in the 'emotional support' dimension *and* a defining principle that can have expression in all the dimensions.

Unfortunately, debates about patients' experiences of care are fraught with language problems: *patient* and *experience* are both problematic. Some commentators dislike *patient* because they see it as positioning the end user in healthcare as subordinate to health professionals and passive. To avoid that association, in mental health services professionals call patients *service users* – but this term too is contested because some service users rightly say, 'There is more to me and more to my life than the fact that I use mental health services.'

A different but related problem is whether to include patients' close others in the frame of reference along with patients, and what to call them. Conventionally, service providers and policymakers refer to close others as *carers*, but the individuals to whom the term applies may not see or wish to see themselves as carers. One alternative is to frame everyone – the patient and the patient's close others – as *consumers*. This is the term of choice in the healthcare systems of Australia and Canada; in the UK, policymakers often use the term, and the newly created Healthwatch organisation describes itself as the national 'consumer champion' in health and social care (Healthwatch, 2014), but the term has little traction with patients, the general public or the NHS.

Experience is also a problematic word. *Patient experience* is a management term and is ungrammatical. The Point of Care Programme (and subsequently the Point of Care Foundation) uses the pragmatic but somewhat unsatisfactory formulation *patients' experiences* as a way of acknowledging that experiences are plural.

Experiences of care are empirical realities: we can collect data about experiences directly from patients and other sources, but *patients' experience* itself is not the goal. The goal may be *patient-centred care, patient- and family-centred care, person-centred care, relationship-centred care* or *personalised care*, but these and other sound-alike terms have subtle but different meanings and appeal to different audiences. Some writers and audiences are conscious that the terms have different meanings, but others are not and use them interchangeably. Faced with these problems, in 2008 the Point of Care Programme commissioned research into reactions to these and other frequently used terms (such as *dignity, respect, compassion* and *humanity*) in four NHS organisations (Wood, 2008).

The research showed that people at every level of the organisations, from non-executive directors to senior clinical staff and porters, found the language confusing and unconvincing. The idea that you might strive to put yourself in the patient's shoes, or to see through the patient's eyes was widely understood, but terms such as *patient-centred, person-centred* and so on were seen as management words or words for the boardroom, not the hospital. Interestingly, some thought *compassion* was an 'extreme' word, relevant perhaps to end-of-life care, but not to everyday and ordinary settings. People at all levels and in all professional groups preferred everyday human words such as *respect, dignity, sensitive, kind, welcoming, friendly* and *comfort* to 'management' words (Wood, 2008).

Latterly, the term *person-centred care* has received more attention. A person-centred service is one where health and social care professionals work collaboratively with people to help them make better-informed decisions and manage their own health and care. This requires a change in behaviour and mindset from healthcare professionals and patients – supported by a system that puts patients at its heart (Health Foundation, 2014). Person-centred care is based on four principles:

1. Affording people dignity, respect and compassion
2. Offering coordinated care, support or treatment
3. Offering personalised care, support or treatment
4. Being enabling (Health Foundation, 2014).

These principles are compatible with the Institute of Medicine definition of *patient-centred care*, but advocates of person-centred care tend to reject the term *patient experience* as positioning patients as passive recipients rather than full participants in their own care (Collins, 2014).

The case person-centred care makes for patient activation and enablement is persuasive. However, the Point of Care Foundation goal remains patient-centred care as defined by the Institute of Medicine. The reasons for sticking with *patient-centred care* are as follows:

➤ It explicitly acknowledges the *multidimensional* nature of patients' experiences.

➤ The 'information, communication and education' dimension can encompass patient activation and enablement.

➤ It defines the dimensions of services for *all* patients, including those who are vulnerable and cannot or will not be enabled to be active.

➤ It focuses on the physical, organisational, relational and transactional elements of care involving *all* staff, not only the subset involving patients and health professionals.

When it started, the aim of the Point of Care Programme was to understand hospital patients' experiences and find out whether there are effective interventions to improve them. Early on in the work, we were persuaded by the strength of the evidence of the positive impact of staff engagement and well-being on patients' experiences (Raleigh et al., 2009; Boorman, 2009) to reframe the aims to include improving staff experience. The evidence of high levels of stress among NHS staff and the relationship between stress, burnout, loss of ideals (Maben et al., 2007) and compassionate care was compelling (Firth-Cozens and Cornwell, 2009) and has become even stronger with the publication of more recent research (Maben et al., 2012).

Improvement

The multidimensional nature of patients' experiences makes identifying how to improve care experiences very challenging. The implications of the relational aspects of most dimensions mean that change is only possible with the cooperation and effort of all staff. Improving patients' experiences is significantly more challenging than improving other dimensions of quality (such as access, for example) where it is possible to achieve results by reorganising activities and processes (the transactional elements) without tackling intrinsic motivation, or than persuading individuals and groups to change their behaviour (the relational aspects).

From the outset, it was important for the Point of Care Programme to learn from quality-improvement initiatives in the UK and elsewhere (Leatherman and Sutherland, 2008). These are the key lessons we took from the literature:

➤ The commitment of senior leaders to the work of improving quality is essential.

➤ Achieving real and sustained improvements in quality of care takes time. Internationally, the healthcare organisations delivering the best care have been working to achieve high-quality care over many years.

➤ Significant and sustained improvements in the quality of healthcare are difficult to achieve. The quantum of improvement made in any single initiative is invariably modest.

➤ Sustained improvement in any aspect of quality only occurs when the priorities, actions and incentives of individuals working at every level of the system are aligned around a common goal. One of the best examples of this in the NHS is the reduction in waiting lists and waiting times achieved over the last decade.

➤ Making change is one thing; making a change that results in improvement is another. Measurement is critically important because it provides the only way to tell the difference between the two.

With these lessons in mind, we turned to the literature on innovation and the spread of good ideas for help with assessing the claims made for different interventions to improve patients' experience of care and/or staff experience (Greenhalgh et al., 2004). Working from the evidence, we developed five criteria to assess interventions for improvement we came across and selected the ones we thought worth replicating, adopting or testing further. The criteria an intervention had to satisfy were as follows:

1. Relevance: The intervention had to be relevant to the multidimensional and complex nature of patients' and/or staff experience because it directly reflected or was compatible with a systems perspective. It was not about one dimension of experience (e.g. physical comfort or communication) and did not involve only one professional group.

2. Describable: It had to be described in enough detail for it to be possible to replicate it somewhere else.

3. Flexible: It had to be flexible and able to be adapted to suit different contexts.

4. Spread: The intervention had to have spread beyond its place of origin to other services and/or organisations.

5. Assessable: It had to have been subject to an external assessment, with evidence from that external assessment available to others.

Using these criteria, we focused on two types of interventions – those designed to have a direct impact on patients' experience of care, experience-based co-design (EBCD) and patient- and family-centred care (PFCC); and those designed to foster conditions in which staff are more likely to respond to patients individually and be supportive (Schwartz Center, n.d.).

Experience based co-design (EBCD) and patient- and family-centred care (PFCC) start from the shared insight that patients and healthcare workers of all kinds 'walk in different shoes' and that any effort to improve patients' experience needs to be based on data detailing their perspectives on care. Staff cannot see the service through the patient's eyes, but they can discover what it is like from a variety of sources, including:

➤ Data from patients' feedback

➤ Complaints and compliments

➤ Conversations (more or less formal and structured) with patients and their close others

➤ Independent observers and mystery shoppers

➤ Films, dramatic productions, poems, music

➤ Structured observations of care

➤ Patient shadowing

➤ Routine administrative data on delays, lengths of stay, and so on.

EBCD and PFCC offer different solutions to the problem of seeing care experiences through the patient's eyes.

Experience-based Co-design (EBCD)

Co-design is a process developed by design professionals to foster collaboration between end users of products (in this case, patients using a particular service) and other stakeholders (health professionals), with the aim of finding solutions to problems in the way the product or service functions. The goal is to achieve a user- rather than a producer-centred service that meets all the technical/clinical requirements of the product *and* satisfies the end user. Co-design and co-production are similar processes, although co-design attaches more weight to the design sciences. In both, there is a commitment to *participatory* or *emancipatory* processes – meaning that everyone with a professional or personal stake in the product or service is treated as having an equal voice and is able to take part in the process.

In co-design, the end users' experience of the product/service is defined as the 'aesthetic'. In the case of an entity as complex as a personal service, the aesthetic is produced by everything that affects the end users' senses: what they see, hear, touch, smell and how they feel while they are in contact with the service. In healthcare, the 'aesthetic' is comprised of these factors:

➤ The physical environment and artefacts (e.g. lighting, flooring, equipment, furniture, posters, paper documents).

➤ Events that do (and do not) occur (e.g. the amount of time patients spend with others versus time alone; the number of staff involved with the same patient at the same time and over time; the number of 'hand-offs' in a care process).

➤ How staff interact with each other and with the patient (e.g. whether staff pass information about the patient on to one another; whether the patient is dressed or undressed in different settings; how patients are handled physically).

➤ The cultural norms of the service – the 'way things get done around here'.

Paul Bate and Glenn Robert, with the NHS Institute for Innovation and Improvement, devised EBCD for a project to improve the quality of service to patients with head and neck cancer at Luton and Dunstable Hospital. Their preferred method for seeing through the patients' eyes was to interview patients, film the interviews and, in collaboration with the patients, edit the hours of footage down into a single film of manageable length that captured the range of experiences in the care journey. They also interviewed but did not film the staff. They brought the patients' film along with the output from staff interviews and maps of the care process to a meeting (the 'co-design event') where patients and staff together reviewed all the materials and collectively agreed the priorities for action. (Full details of the methodology are available on the King's Fund website at www.kingsfund.org.uk/projects/ebcd.)

Since 2007, EBCD methods have been adopted in the NHS and around the world, and a simpler and equally effective version that avoids the need to make the patient films from scratch, instead using 'trigger films' from the substantial archive at HealthTalkOnline, has been developed (Locock et al., 2014). The evidence from EBCD projects demonstrates that

➤ with careful management and expert facilitation, patients and staff can overcome anxieties about each other and collaborate together as equals;

➤ they can identify the 'touch points' (also known as the 'moments of truth') in the course of a care journey, which are the moments that resonate especially strongly for patients or staff, either positively or negatively;

➤ they can use the touch points to prioritise improvements – enhancing positive touch points and eliminating the negative touch points;

➤ co-design working groups involving patients and staff can implement changes using standard improvement methods;

➤ the act of patients and staff working together serves as a dynamic catalyst for change and has a dramatic impact on staff motivation;

➤ participants from both groups report that the process itself transforms their view of what is possible in a lasting way. Patients say they prefer working with staff to recording their opinions in surveys or focus groups. Staff say they feel reinvigorated and able to work in the way they had imagined when they first started work with patients.

Patient and Family-centred Care (PFCC)

PFCC originated in the Pittsburgh University Medical Center, where orthopaedic surgeon Tony di Gioia sought an holistic method that would improve clinical outcomes and patient satisfaction without increasing costs (PFCC Innovation Center, 2014). The Point of Care adapted his PFCC guide for UK audiences, added a focus on staff experience and training in the fundamentals of quality improvement and ran two waves of an improvement collaborative with 25 front-line teams from

16 English NHS trusts and Welsh Health Boards. The aim was to achieve improvements in the services provided by the participating teams and increase the capability of the host Trusts and Boards to deliver patient and family-centred care.

PFCC is a six-step process for transforming a care experience from the current state to an ideal state. A care experience is the sequence of events and processes in the delivery of care as seen through the patient's eyes. Instead of filming interviews with patients, data on patients' care experiences are collected by members of staff who shadow patients from the beginning of the care experience through to the end. The insights from shadowing are combined with data collected from patient interviews and other routinely available sources (patient surveys, complaints, administrative and performance data, safety data, staff surveys) to understand the quality of the care experiences and decide (numerical) improvement goals. Once the goals are clear, the team develops a logic tree, using a mechanism known as a driver diagram to analyse the primary and secondary drivers of the phenomenon they wish to change. As in EBCD, small, project-based-change working groups, ideally formed of patients and staff working together, then work on the selected improvement areas, using the standard improvement methods. Full details of the methodology, with examples of driver diagrams, are available on the King's Fund website at www.kingsfund.org.uk/projects/pfcc.

The majority of teams participating in the two PFCC collaboratives achieved measureable improvements in patients' care experiences. Patient shadowing has a lasting impact on the staff who do it because it makes them aware – often for the first time – of the critical importance of the relational dimensions of experience. For example at Great Ormond Street, the team working with boys suffering from Duchenne muscular dystrophy changed the way they organised the outpatient clinics to make the process smoother, less tiring and less stressful for the boys and their families; improved the way they communicated with families (e.g. texting when results were available); and made improvements in the physical environment to afford the patients more privacy. Families and staff reported improved clinic organisation, and better care planning. At Alder Hey Hospital, the team focused on children with acute abdominal pain in the Emergency Department. Here, the staff who shadowed patients discovered that the processes they had thought were in place to give children immediate pain relief when they arrived in the department were not working well and that it was taking a long time (sometimes hours) for the child to be assessed. As a result of their work, the team saw that they needed to encourage the children (and the adults accompanying the children) to 'speak up' when children were in pain so that staff would know there was a problem. By telling the stories of individual children to their colleagues in the radiology and surgical departments, they were able to speed up the diagnostic process so that children who needed surgery could be operated on more quickly, and children who did not need surgery could be sent home. One of the most significant changes that came about was the surgeons' decision to 'ring-fence' four beds specifically so that they could attend to the children with acute abdominal pain very quickly.

EBCD and PFCC address a key problem in all modern healthcare systems, which is that, although staff may want to provide the best care possible, most organisations and front-line teams find it difficult to walk in the patients' shoes and do not know what they can do to improve patients' experiences. Staff may believe they understand patients' experiences of care, but this is not necessarily the case, and methods that enable them to see care through patients' eyes are powerful and transformative (Hawkes, 2013).

The key messages from EBCD and PFCC are the same. Sustained improvement in patients' experience requires the following:

1. Active and committed leadership must come from executive directors who invest their own time in working with the teams and use what they learn to develop the organisation's corporate capacity to improve patients' experiences.

2. Medical leadership must be provided by doctors who actively involve themselves in shadowing patients and co-design activities. Doctors have a disproportionate influence on the culture of services and multidisciplinary staff groups. When senior doctors actively endorse efforts to improve patients' experiences, the work proceeds faster and goes further; when they stand back from it, it has less reach and eventually falters.

3. An infrastructure must exist to support the application of the improvement effort by providing help collecting patient-based data and clear links to other improvement projects and existing priorities.

4. Time for staff to carry out improvement work must be provided.

5. A focus should be placed on the lived, direct experience of patients and families.

6. And ideally, patients and family must be involved.

What prevents improvement happening is the absence of the factors listed above and the adverse influence of other key contextual factors, including these:

1. The external and political context in which organisations operate – the level of stability, local structural changes within the health economy, local priorities.

2. Whether there is an organisational imperative behind the work which brings the attention and support of senior leaders.

3. The pressure of work and demands on the system – if it is out of balance with the level of resources for long periods of time it will overwhelm improvement efforts.

4. Local front-line team stability.

5. Strong relationships inside the organisation.

Interventions Designed to Support Staff in Their Work with Patients

In the early days of the Point of Care programme, the compelling evidence that staff experience shapes patients' experiences of care made us look for effective interventions to support staff in their work with patients and drew us to Schwartz Rounds.

Schwartz Center Rounds

Schwartz Center Rounds were originally developed as an intervention to strengthen relationships between caregivers and patients by the Boston-based, not-for-profit Schwartz Center for Compassionate Healthcare. In 2009, the King's Fund (via the Point of Care programme) made an agreement with the Schwartz Center to pilot Rounds in two NHS acute hospital trusts – the first expansion of Rounds internationally. Today, the Point of Care Foundation is the sole licensed provider of training and support to organisations wishing to run Schwartz Rounds in the UK and as of December 2014 had helped over 90 NHS trusts and hospices introduce the Rounds.

The Schwartz Center and the Rounds are named after Kenneth Schwartz, an American lawyer who was diagnosed with terminal lung cancer in his forties. In the course of his treatment, Kenneth discovered that the 'smallest acts of kindness' on the part of healthcare professionals could make 'the unbearable bearable' for patients. 'If I have learned anything,' he wrote, 'it is that we never know when, how or whom a serious illness will strike. If and when it does, each one of us wants not simply the best possible care for our body but for our whole being' (www.theschwartzcenter. org/media/patient_story.pdf).

A round is a simple intervention: it is a confidential one-hour-long meeting at which staff from different disciplines discuss the relational aspects of their work with patients with each other. In contrast to traditional 'Grand Rounds', which are teaching sessions where doctors present the medical problems and treatment of particular patients to medical audiences, a Schwartz Round is about the human (not the clinical) aspects of the care and is open to *all* staff. Typical topics discussed at Schwartz Rounds, for example, would be 'a patient I will never forget'; 'when is enough (care) enough?'; and 'when the patient and family members disagree'.

The evaluations of the Rounds in the United States and in the UK (Lown and Manning, 2010; Goodrich, 2012) show they have a positive impact on participating staff, staff beliefs about patient care, teamwork, perceptions of levels of stress and support in the workplace and changes in institutional practices and policies. The findings demonstrate that following rounds, participants reported better teamwork and less stress. Rounds also enhanced participants' likelihood of attending to psychosocial and emotional aspects of care and enhanced their beliefs about the importance of empathy (Goodrich, 2012). Furthermore, the impact of rounds on these outcomes increased in line with the number of participants who attended. The evidence suggests that Schwartz Rounds provide an important space for staff to share the highs and lows of their work and gain support and insights from colleagues (Lown and Manning, 2010; Goodrich, 2012). The assumption is that this in turn influences relationships both between colleagues and with patients and ultimately the delivery of better patient care.

The impact of the Schwartz Rounds in healthcare settings in England is now being evaluated with a final report from the study scheduled for publication in late 2016.

The Changing Context and Reflections on the Future

Since 2010, the impact of devastating reports of failures in the care of older people in hospitals and residential and nursing care homes, the report of the Public Inquiry into the Mid Staffordshire Foundation NHS Trust 2013 (Francis, 2013) and the public exposure of criminal neglect and brutality towards residents with learning disabilities at Winterbourne View Hospital (South Gloucestershire Adults Safeguarding Board, 2012) has ensured political and media interest in the quality of care has been sustained.

It is unlikely that patient safety or patient experience will slip down the priority list, although that does not mean to say that it is not important to be vigilant – anything is possible. In the UK, there is a strong sense of a gathering momentum, linking together different groups of academics, health professionals, patient leaders and other activists for change, through social media and in the real world. Elsewhere, and without the catalyst of Mid Staffordshire or Winterbourne View, similar things are happening. In the United States, Canada, Australia and some European countries, the call for transformation in the culture of health services, support for patients' active involvement in their own care and decisions about services are increasing. It is interesting to consider why this is happening everywhere. Perhaps it has something to do with the crisis in acute medicine and the failure to respond adequately to the needs of large numbers of people living with multiple long-term conditions. Or perhaps it is due to rising expectations and patients' and caregivers' refusal to tolerate not being treated as a person.

For all this activity, patients' experience of care still lags behind the other dimensions of quality – in terms of investment in research, practical tools and techniques for improvement, and education. It has not yet attracted the political or professional attention it deserves. Perhaps this should not surprise us as it represents a much more radical challenge to the status quo than action on the other dimensions of quality, all of which can be accommodated within existing power structures. However, the momentum is growing, and if nurses come to appreciate that it is possible to work with patients in a different way and to derive more not less satisfaction, it can succeed.

References

Adamson, E., B. Dewar, J. H. Donaldson, M. Gentleman, M. Gray, D. Horsburgh, L. King et al. (2012) *Leadership in Compassionate Care Programme Final Report* (Edinburgh: Napier University).

Bate, P. and G. Robert (2007) *Bringing User Experience to Healthcare Improvement* (Oxford: Radcliffe).

Boorman, S. (2009) NHS Health and Well-Being Final Report, www.orderonline. dh.gov.uk.

Chochinov, H. M. (2007) 'Dignity and the Essence of Medicine: The A, B, C, and D of Dignity Conserving Care', *British Medical Journal*, 335: 184–7.

Collins, A. (2014) *Measuring What Really Matters. Towards a Coherent Measurement System to Support Person-centred Care* (London: The Health Foundation).

Coulter, A., R. Fitzpatrick and J. Cornwell (2009) *Measures of Patients' Experience in Hospital: Purpose, Method and Uses* (London: The King's Fund).

Delbanco, T. L. (1996) 'Quality of Care through the Patient's Eyes', *British Medical Journal*, 313: 832–3.

Department of Health (DH) (2008) *High Quality Care for All – NHS Next Stage Review final report* (London: DH).

Dr Foster Limited (2010) *Patient Experience,* The Intelligent Board 2010 (London: Dr Foster).

Firth-Cozens, J. and J. Cornwell (2009) *Enabling Compassionate Care in Acute Hospital Settings* (London: The King's Fund).

Francis, R. (2013) 'The Mid Staffordshire NHS Foundation Trust public inquiry', www.midstaffspublicinquiry.com/sites/default/files/report/Executive%20summary.pdf, accessed 4 August 2014.

Goodrich, J. (2012) 'Supporting Hospital Staff to Provide Compassionate Care: Do Schwartz Center Rounds Work in English Hospitals?', *Journal of the Royal Society of Medicine*, 105(3): 117–22. doi: 10.1258/jrsm.2011.110183.

Goodrich, J. and J. Cornwell (2008) 'Seeing the Person in the Patient', The Point of Care review paper (London: The King's Fund).

Greenhalgh, T., G. Robert, F. MacFarlane, P. Bate and O. Kyriakidou (2004) 'Diffusion of Innovations in Service Organizations: Systematic Review and Recommendations', *Milbank Quarterly*, 82(4): 581–629.

Hawkes, N. (2013) 'Patients' Actual Care Pathways Often Differ Markedly from Doctors' Perceptions', *British Medical Journal*, 347: f6728.

The Health Foundation (2014) 'What Is Person-Centred Care?', www.health.org.uk/areas-of-work/topics/person-centred-care/person-centred-care/, accessed 4 August 2014.

Healthwatch (2014) 'The National Consumer Champion in Health and Social Care', www.healthwatch.co.uk, accessed 25 July 2014.

iWantGreatCare; www.iwantgreatcare.org, accessed 27 April 2016.

Institute of Medicine (1999) *To Err is Human: Building a Safer Health System* (Washington, DC: National Academy Press).

Institute of Medicine (2001) *Crossing the Quality Chasm: A New Health System for the 21st Century* (Washington, DC: National Academy Press).

The King's Fund (2014) 'Patient and Family-Centred Care Toolkit', www.kingsfund.org.uk/projects/pfcc/, accessed 4 August 2014.

The King's Fund (2013) 'Experience-based Co-design Toolkit', 4 December, www.kingsfund.org.uk/projects/ebcd/, accessed 4 August 2014.

Leatherman, S. and K. Sutherland (2008) *The Quest for Quality in the NHS: Refining the NHS Reforms* (London: Nuffield Trust).

Locock, L., G. Robert, A. Boaz, S. Vougioukalou, C. Shuldham, J. Fielden, S. Ziebland et al. (2014). 'Testing Accelerated Experience-Based Co-Design: A Qualitative Study of Using a National Archive of Patient Experience Narrative Interviews to Promote Rapid Patient-Centred Service Improvement', *Health Services and Delivery Research*, 2(4): 1–150.

Lown, B. and C. Manning (2010) 'The Schwartz Center Rounds: Evaluation of an Interdisciplinary Approach to Enhancing Patient-Centered Communication, Teamwork and Provider Support', *Academic Medicine,* 85(6): 1073–81.

Maben, J., S. Latter and J. Macleod Clark (2007) 'The Sustainability of Ideals, Values and the Nursing Mandate: Evidence from a Longitudinal Qualitative Study', *Nursing Inquiry*, 14(2): 99–113.

Maben, J., R. Peccei, M. Adams, G. Robert, A. Richardson, T. Murrells and E. Morrow (2012) 'Exploring the Relationship between Patients' Experiences of Care and the Influence of Staff Motivation, Affect and Wellbeing', National Institute for Health Research Service Delivery and Organisation Programme.

Mylod, D. E. and T. H. Lee (2013) 'A Framework for Reducing Suffering in Healthcare', http://blogs.hbr.org/2013/11/a-framework-for-reducing-suffering-in-health-care/, accessed 30 July 2014.

National Quality Board and Department of Health (2011) 'NHS Patient Experience Framework', www.gov.uk/government/uploads/system/uploads/attachment_data/file/215159/dh_132788.pdf, accessed 4 August 2014.

NHS Institute Worldwide (2014) 'The Productive Ward', www.institute.nhs.uk/international/general/the_productive_ward.html, accessed 28 July 2014.

PFCC Innovation Center (2014) 'What is PFCC?', www.pfcc.org/what-is-pfcc, accessed 4 August 2014.

Picker Institute; http://pickerinstitute.org/, accessed 27 April 2016.

Planetree; www.planetree.org, accessed 27 April 2016.

Raleigh, V.S., D. Hussey, I. Seccombe and R. Qi (2009) 'Do Associations between Staff and Inpatient Feedback Have the Potential for Improving Patient Experience? An Analysis of Surveys in NHS Acute Trusts in England', *Quality and Safety in Healthcare*, 18: 347–54.

Redfern, S., C. Normand, S. Christian, A. Gilmore, T. Murrells, I. Norman and W. Stevens (1997) 'An Evaluation of Nursing Development Units', *Journal of Research in Nursing*, 2(4): 292–303. doi: 10.1177/174498719700200410.

Robert, G. and J. Cornwell (2011) 'What Matters to Patients? Developing the Evidence Base for Measuring and Improving Patient Experience Project Report', www.wales.nhs.uk/sites3/Documents/420/Final%20Project%20Report%20pdf%20doc%20january%202012%20%282%29.pdf, accessed 3 August 2014.

South Gloucestershire Adults Safeguarding Board (2012) 'Serious Case Review: Winterbourne View Hospital', www.southglos.gov.uk/health-and-social-care/care-for-adults/safeguarding-vulnerable-adults/winterbourne-view/, accessed 26 July 2014.

The Schwartz Center for Compassionate Healthcare (n.d.), www.theschwartzcenter.org/supporting-caregivers, accessed 14 August 2014.

Wood, V. (2008) 'The King's Fund – "The Point of Care": A Report on the Findings of Qualitative Research among Healthcare Professionals', unpublished report, available on request from the Point of Care Foundation.

8

The Emotional Labour of Nursing

Yvonne Sawbridge

Introduction

Nursing in the UK has been subject to intense scrutiny and criticism in the wake of the Francis Public Inquiry (2010, 2013) into poor care at Mid Staffordshire NHS Foundation Trust. The public, media-led narrative largely focused on individual accountability ('good/bad' nurse); the move to degree-level nurse education ('too clever to care') and some contextual issues – staffing numbers and workload for example. The introduction to this book explored a range of factors that can contribute to the delivery of poor nursing care, which takes the discussion beyond blaming the individual nurse. While not ignoring the responsibility of individuals to deliver good care, this chapter focuses on a specific concept which is rarely discussed in the debate about poor care: the role of emotional labour in the delivery of compassionate care. It describes the concept of emotional labour in more detail, explores the relevant literature and considers its implications for the nursing workforce and compassionate care. The chapter also reports the learning from an action research project conducted in three hospital trusts to implement an emotional support system for staff, in partnership with the Samaritans organisation (a charity which provides a confidential listening service for people in distress). The project involved the adaptation of a model of support used by the Samaritans organisation (see Box 8.1) for their volunteers and highlighted the complexities of developing appropriate support systems for staff in hospital settings. Despite concluding that it was not feasible to adapt this system for a ward environment, the project raised the awareness of emotional labour and led to further work in this area.

Context

Francis (2010, 2013) provides a compelling and distressing narrative from families and carers of patients who experienced appalling care. The report demonstrates that some nurses did not fulfil their professional responsibilities and failed to act in a caring and considerate manner.

A crucial question, therefore, is what went wrong? The current negative coverage of nurses and nursing in the press creates a difficult background against which to explore the issues openly and honestly, and identify what needs to change. This coverage generally takes a simplistic, often blaming view (Marrin, 2009) rather than engaging with some of the wider issues such as the complexities of the care environment. The lack of recognition that patients in hospital are sicker, require more time and have more complex needs is overlooked in the simplistic characterisations of poor care. The issues of the community nursing workforce captured in the Queen's Nursing Institute Report (2014) in terms of reductions in district nurse training, organisational upheaval and workload pressures are similarly ignored. It is easier to blame uncaring nurses (Odone, 2011) than to tackle the endemic organisational barriers to good care. Although poor care cannot be condoned, it is not unreasonable to call for a more informed analysis of the issues. An understanding of the reality of caring is needed if solutions are to be found.

It was this concern that prompted a more reflective approach to the issues uncovered and a desire to move beyond the headlines, to try to understand the underlying cause of this poor care. The recognition that the organisational context can result in 'good' people delivering poor care (Iles, 2011) suggested that the reasons for this needed further exploration. We convened a 'think tank' of six chief nurses to explore the issues; it reviewed the literature and identified three themes – nurse education, the environment of care and the emotional labour of care (Sawbridge and Hewison, 2011). The latter theme has received relatively little attention in the recent debates about compassionate care and is the focus of this chapter.

What Is Emotional Labour?

The term *physical labour* is understood to mean hard physical effort and is often accounted for in management practice. For example lifting patients is viewed as a physical risk for staff (and patients), and so organisations take responsibility for the provision of equipment on wards or in patients' homes. If they failed in this duty, then they would understand if the Health and Safety Executive called them to account. However, emotional labour is less well recognised, does not attract the same level of management support and is rarely discussed in practice.

Emotional labour means that there are work-appropriate emotions which need to be displayed, depending on the work role, and these may differ from the emotions an individual may feel. In addition, you need to elicit an appropriate emotional response in your client/patient/customer. Hochschild (1983) first coined the phrase *emotional labour* in her study of air stewards working for American Airlines. She was interested in the emotions employees were expected to display as part of their paid labour. (Her work is discussed in more detail in Chapter 11.) She defined it as 'an induction or suppression of feeling in order to sustain an outward appearance that produces in others a sense of being cared for' (p. 7).

Pam Smith in her research into the emotional labour of nursing (Smith, 1992, 2012) concludes that nursing is a profession which involves considerable emotional labour as a *role requirement*. This is an important concept, as it denotes this as something that should feature on the person specification and job description – just as driving would be a role requirement for a chauffeur for example. Recognition of this then naturally redirects the focus of attention from the deeds of the individual per se to the duty of the employing organisation in recruiting, developing and supporting nurses who are able to deliver this core element of their role.

Mastracci et al. (2012; also see Chapter 11) describe emotional labour as a requirement of a quality public service and expand the definition to describe three key elements: having direct contact with the public (face-to-face or on the telephone); producing an emotional state in this person; and presenting a role-appropriate emotion at that time, even if this entails a suppression of one's own emotions.

These three elements of emotional labour can be seen in nursing. For example the nurse who is actively working to reduce the anxiety of a patient waiting to undergo a serious operation, but also reliving the experience of her own mother who had a similar operation and did not survive; or dealing with unpleasant bodily fluids while portraying a calm, caring and matter-of-fact demeanour. Nurses need to both reduce anxiety in the patient and display a sense of calm professionalism, regardless of their own underlying emotions. This can be exacting.

Nurses often deal with distress, tragedy, death and dying. This is not a typical working experience for most people, and the impact of this on the health and well-being of nurses needs to be recognised. Menzies (1960) identified nurses as fulfilling the primary purpose of the hospital as they are the only members of the workforce who 'must provide continuous care for patients, day and night, all the year round' (p. 97). She concluded, 'Nurses are confronted with the threat and the reality of suffering and death as few lay people are. Their work involves carrying out tasks which, by ordinary standards, are distasteful, disgusting and frightening.'

This is a truth which is rarely discussed. Nurses do not usually voice the way they feel about unpleasant tasks, such as dealing with bodily fluids – possibly in order to protect patients from any embarrassment or concern. However, care must be provided as if there is no emotional cost to the nurse – hence the need for hard emotional labour, as a role requirement for nurses.

Emotional Labour in Practice

Although there have been many changes in nursing since Menzies (1960) conducted her work, the demands of caring have not diminished, and emotions including anger and anxiety continue to feature in nurses' work (Waddington and Fletcher, 2005). Aside from the toll of providing direct care, nurses have expressed feelings of frustration and anger about cost containment measures and managerial strategies which prevent them from delivering the best care to their patients (Bone, 2002). Moving an elderly patient out of hospital late at night to accommodate admissions from A&E would be an example of this. The nurse has both a duty of care to his or her individual patient and a responsibility as an employee to fulfil the priorities of the organisation. When these are in tension, as in this situation, it compounds the levels of emotional labour nurses are required to deliver. This has an impact on the ability of staff to provide compassionate care for patients; if their 'emotional bank account' is overdrawn, they may have nothing left to give.

Maben et al. (2012) found strong links between staff well-being and patient outcomes, and recommended that supporting staff with the emotional aspects of care was an important area to address. This complements Smith's work (2012) and highlights that the impact of emotional labour is more widespread than just having an effect on the well-being of an individual nurse. It is also an important element of patient care and a legitimate concern for any organisation responsible for delivering compassionate care.

For those involved in emotional labour, there are positive and negative consequences. Caring for someone effectively can bring a sense of fulfilment and satisfaction (Bolton and Boyd, 2003). However, if the pressures are relentless and nurses are unable to provide the care they see as crucial, then emotional labour can take its toll. Gray and Smith (2009) highlight the invisibility of emotion in nursing and suggest that the constant suppression of powerful emotions is likely to affect practitioners sufficiently to cause burnout. Leiter and Maslach (1988) described burnout as having three components: emotional exhaustion, depersonalisation and reduced sense of personal accomplishment, which can result in 'a shift from the positive and caring to the negative and uncaring' (Maslach, 2003: 27). This has a direct impact on patient care. Nurses may stop hearing the call bells, or avoid looking up from the nurses' station despite an obvious queue of relatives. Community staff may focus on the task rather than engage more meaningfully in their patients' lives. Peate's (2014), editorial, concluded: 'When there is stress, often confounded by staffing problems and lack of teamwork and support, then this stress accumulates until the care giver just detaches emotionally from his or her work. The nurse is delivering care but may not even be cognisant of what he or she is doing as a result of the stress' (p. 251).

One of the features of emotional labour is its invisibility. The patient must not see the 'surface acting' (Hochschild, 1983) that this emotion work entails, and a passer-by would merely witness a conversation, not understand the true nature of the effort taking place. This means it is rarely taken account of in management practice. For example Rowland (2014) identified that ambulance staff used a variety of coping mechanisms to deal with issues they face in their working day. They would use their time in between calls to debrief in an informal and unstructured way, using humour or anecdotes, though they may not have understood the role this played in terms of supporting each other and 'managing' emotional labour. However, in order to meet shorter response times (targets), managers placed ambulance staff in 'standby locations', geographically placed across the 'patch', rather than at a central ambulance station, meaning they had most areas covered. This removed the opportunities to return to base between calls, and meant that some staff felt more stressed and said they were taking more time off sick. A recent report (Melley, 2014) identified an increased attrition rate, with 1015 paramedics leaving their job in 2013–14, compared with 593 in the same period two years earlier. The unintended consequence of the organisation's approach to meeting response time targets was the removal of an important support mechanism from their staff – albeit that it was never understood or described in this way, least of all by staff.

Emotional Labour Today

Building on the example of changing practices for ambulance staff noted above, changes in nursing practice and rituals may have exacerbated the negative impact of emotional labour on nurses. For example, although it had limitations, 'task allocation' provided a means of maintaining a level of emotional detachment and protection from an overwhelming anxiety (Menzies, 1960). Carrying out a series of discrete tasks, such as taking the temperatures of all patients in a ward, provided a focus on the task, not the patient, thus reducing levels of emotional involvement. With the introduction of the nursing process (a problem-solving approach to delivering individualised care), work was organised on the basis of patient allocation rather than task assignment, with an associated emphasis on caring for the patient as an individual (Smith, 1992: 39). Although there are likely benefits for patients, this brought concurrent demands in terms of emotional labour. A reciprocal increase in emotional support might enable these interactions to remain therapeutic and compassionate – but this needs to be recognised.

Other changes in working practice may have removed routines and practices that served as coping strategies for nurses in the past. These include changes in the handover of patients to oncoming staff. Once these handovers took place in an office and may have provided a respite for staff to share their 'vocabularies of complaint' (Turner, 1987) and provide them with a safe space to vent their feelings. Many now take place at the bedside rather than in an office (Sawbridge and Hewison, 2011), in full view of patients, and allow no scope for sharing of emotions in private. Community staff have similarly experienced changes in working practice and are increasingly expected to be 'agile workers', meaning that they are working alone throughout the day, and discouraged from returning to base at lunchtime, limiting the opportunity for them to have a safe space in which to 'sound off' about the demands of their work. 'Talking shop' (Guy, Newman and Mastracci, 2008), sharing 'vocabularies of complaint' (Turner, 1987) and 'gossiping' (Waddington and Fletcher, 2005) in private are all important ways of managing emotional labour, and it appears many of these have been eroded.

Other changes include the closure of on-site hospital laundries and staff changing rooms preventing staff from having the opportunity to 'step out' of their work role, symbolised by leaving their uniform at work. In addition the pressure on hospital estates has resulted in staff rooms being converted into clinical rooms and staff canteens being closed, meaning staff take their breaks with visitors. This loss of protected space where staff can meet *without* patients or carers being present is likely to make it harder for nurses to manage their emotional labour.

This may be compounded by a lack of resources (staff or equipment). For example there are 40 per cent fewer district nurses now than there were 15 years ago (NHS Alliance, 2014), and the Safe Staffing Alliance (Osborne, 2014) has collated national and international evidence and concluded that care is compromised on most shifts where there are more than eight patients to one registered nurse – yet 45 per cent of nurses reported looking after more than eight patients when surveyed.

Working to meet competing priorities can also be draining. A community nurse, with a full caseload, may need to create some space for an extra visit for someone needing urgent terminal care. Deciding which of the patients on the caseload can manage without the planned visit in order to accommodate this may prove too difficult. Nurses in this position may either work extra hours (RCN, 2013a, 2013b; The Press Association, 2015) or disappoint a patient expecting a visit, meaning they may leave work without fulfilling the role as they would have wished. Either scenario exacts an emotional toll.

Nurses are constantly involved in high-demand work which they have little control over, and this contributes to their feelings of guilt, low morale and frustration because it impairs their ability to offer good patient care (Maben et al., 2012). If nurses do not have support for caring activities, they may employ strategies to actively disengage from the nurse–patient relationship to protect themselves (Bridges et al., 2012). Their emotional labour becomes too much to bear.

Recognising and responding to this may provide some insight into factors which may affect the individual nurses' ability to deliver compassionate care consistently.

Why Is Emotional Labour Important?

The case for supporting nurses with their emotion work goes beyond the moral imperative of caring for staff, important though that is. It is an underpinning factor in creating the delivery of compassionate care to patients. Although the chair of the CQC stated, 'Kindness and compassion costs nothing'(CQC, 2011), the reality is that it costs a great deal in terms of emotional labour. Crawford and Gilbert (2011) describe compassion as 'a sensitivity to the suffering of others with a deep commitment to try and relieve it' (p. 2). It differs to kindness in that being kind is usually a pleasant act – giving a gift or collecting someone's shopping – whereas compassion can be unpleasant as it requires an engagement with someone's distress or suffering. Cole-King and Gilbert (2011) identify the need for awareness and engagement as well as skilled intervention and action. As noted earlier in this chapter, those staff 'running on empty' in terms of their 'emotional bank account' may develop an unhealthy detachment and therefore not notice the distress of others. Even if they do notice this distress, they may feel at risk of feeling overwhelmed, and therefore turn away from it. This clearly impedes their ability to deliver compassionate care.

Indeed the nursing workforce is showing signs of distress. In an RCN employment survey (2013a), 29 per cent of nurses cited stress or workload as a reason for looking for a new post; 60 per cent work in excess of their contracted hours (increased from 2011), and 18 per cent have other paid jobs to help them meet their financial commitments; 55 per cent of respondents stated that levels of registered nurses had decreased compared to 48 per cent in 2011; and 60 per cent had considered leaving their job in the last 12 months. Thirty-one per cent reported they had been bullied or harassed by a team member or manager in the previous 12 months, and 37 per cent experienced harassment or violence from a patient/client or a relative. Furthermore, the intense pressure on nurses' time results in them rationing care. In a more recent study, it was reported 86 per cent of nurses reported that at least one of the 13 care activities which they consider necessary was left 'undone' on their last shift because of a lack of time (Ball et al., 2014). It is hard to imagine that nurses feel the sense of fulfilment and satisfaction Bolton and Boyd (2003) describe as concomitant with well-being, when they are practising in these circumstances.

Compounding this is the focus on quantitative performance measures and the negative consequences of failure to achieve targets. Youngson (2012) stated:

> When health professionals are abused and de-humanised by an uncaring system, how can we expect them to show compassion to their patients? There's only so much distress professionals can bear and there comes a point where emotional detachment is the only survival strategy. (p. 41)

From the literature, therefore, it can be argued that organisations which require emotional labour to be delivered have a legal responsibility to protect their employees from the risks to their well-being associated with this requirement. Any building site provides a visual reminder of how construction organisations address some of the risks involved for their employees: hard yellow hats are mandatory for example. Protecting nurses from the emotional demands of their role requires a similar concerted effort. Indeed, a report by the Health Safety and Wellbeing Partnership Group (2013) makes this requirement clear: 'The organisation works with staff to develop and implement solutions to manage the stressors in the workplace to reduce, as far as is possible, their effect on staff' (p. 63). Emotional labour is a clear, though poorly addressed, stressor which needs to be managed.

In a study of staff well-being conducted at King's College London it was found that

> that patient experiences are better when staff feel they have a good working environment, support from co-workers and their manager and low emotional exhaustion. These findings are significant and demonstrate that staff wellbeing is an antecedent, not a consequence, of patient care performance. Thus seeking systematically to enhance staff wellbeing is not only important in its own right

but also for the quality of patient experiences. High performing organisations are recognising this and are acting upon staff experience feedback as well as patient experiences of care – seeking to directly improve staff experience as part of quality improvement initiatives. (kcl.ac.uk, 2012)

Finding ways to support nurses to 'top up' their 'emotional bank account' regularly, in order to be capable of delivering the emotional labour which underpins good patient care, is an important management responsibility. A model designed to enable this to happen is explored in the next section.

Time to Care?

In order to discover more about how best to support staff in this aspect of their practice, the feasibility of introducing a model of support in busy hospital wards was explored. The introduction of a model of support which has been used by the Samaritans organisation for over 50 years was the focus of an action research project designed to support staff in practice (Sawbridge and Hewison, 2014).

The Samaritans provide a confidential listening service, available 24/7, 365 days of the year. They have 18,750 volunteers across 201 branches, and it was the model of support they use for their volunteers, rather than the service they provide to callers, which was of particular interest. The well-being of the volunteers is central to the ethos and organisation of the Samaritans. The level of emotional distress callers (and therefore volunteers) experience is often very high – for example some callers are in the act of suicide and want to talk to someone as they die. Clearly this is an extremely difficult task for volunteers, and the Samaritans recognise the emotional impact this work has on volunteers and provide a structured support system for them (see Box 8.1 for a description of this model).

To test the feasibility of applying this model in a hospital environment, an action research project was designed (Hart and Bond, 1995; Bowling, 2002) which included a survey (pre- and post-implementation) to assess staff well-being (ASSET tool) and qualitative interviews with staff to examine their experience of the approach.

The six ward teams were selected by the nurse directors of the partner organisations, and briefing meetings were held to ensure all those involved understood the aims of the project and the level of commitment required. Training was provided for each team member and consisted of theoretical and applied learning in communication, particularly listening, summarising and reflecting skills. It also enabled participants to consider their own emotional needs with regard to care. The Samaritans have developed a structure for the staff training, known as 'The Listening

---

Box 8.1 **The Samaritans' Model of Staff Support**

➤ Each volunteer undergoes a period of training prior to taking calls.

➤ Each shift is between three and five hours, and the volunteers work in pairs as 'buddies'.

➤ The callers are often in a highly distressed state, and the volunteers are actively encouraged to share the last call with their partner in the 'downtimes' in between calls.

➤ If the volunteer needs longer to debrief, the telephones will be turned off to enable this to happen. (It is rare that this action is required as most debriefs are possible in a few minutes.) However, it signifies the importance that the organisation gives to the emotional support of volunteers. They recognise that if the carer isn't cared for, then he or she can't care for the callers, and by this action they demonstrate that they really mean this.

➤ At the end of each shift, the volunteer 'offloads' to the shift leader. This process involves a summary of the types of calls taken by the volunteer *and* how the volunteer is feeling.

➤ The leader will make a judgement about the emotional health of the volunteer, and if the leader feels the volunteer was particularly affected, the leader will call the volunteer the next day to see how he or she is doing.

Wheel', which includes key communication skills such as reflecting, clarifying and summarising. Some of the practical activities, centred on listening and expressing feelings, proved to be challenging for some of the participants, who reported much of their communication on a day-to-day basis was focused on extracting information from patients and colleagues in order to address and solve a series of problems. The emotional support model used by the Samaritans is reliant on staff having highly developed listening skills, so the training was an essential part of the project plan. Those who attended the training reported the time spent developing these skills was valuable (Sawbridge and Hewison, 2014). The training day concluded with the teams producing action plans for the development of ward-based support systems.

It was envisaged that these support systems would follow the Samaritans' approach and involve some 'buddying up' of staff on each shift so a focus on caring for each other, as well as patients, could be incorporated into normal working practices. The intention was that it would be a way of 'being with' each other rather than needing to take time out, given the difficulties of releasing staff from patient care.

Findings

The adoption of the Samaritans' model of staff support in the acute wards proved to be difficult to achieve. Indeed, only three wards completed the project, and only two nurses completed the post-intervention survey; and a further two participated in a follow-up interview to explore their experiences of participating in the project. The lack of data meant that arriving at definitive conclusions concerning the feasibility of adapting the Samaritans' model for use in the NHS was not possible. The report captures the learning from this work, and makes recommendations for future work (Sawbridge and Hewison, 2014). These are explored further below.

The main challenge can be summarised in a comment made by a team member at a ward meeting: 'We don't have time to care.' Staff reported that the workload pressures they were experiencing and low staffing levels meant they were unable to put a staff support system into practice, because they were too busy, despite recognising the need for one. This was compounded in one of the wards by the introduction of 12-hour shifts during the course of the project. Adjusting to new working patterns delayed progress considerably. Even without these difficulties, simply organising one training session took 12 months at one site because the ward team was busy and senior staff had difficulties providing 'backfill' nursing staff to enable the team to attend (despite funding for this being part of the project budget). The absence of active facilitation by senior managers contributed to a lack of momentum in behaviour change once the initial training sessions had been conducted.

Reflections

There were a number of confounding factors which added to the complexity of adapting this model to a ward environment.

Protected Space

It was difficult to find a room on the wards for staff to have space to have a conversation with each other or the Samaritans as part of the project development. The staff room, where one existed, was usually busy, as was the sister's office. When talking to staff, the sluice was often the only place where it was possible to have an uninterrupted conversation. This is in direct contrast to the environment necessary for Samaritans to provide their service, in which volunteers are provided with protected and appropriate space in which to meet with each other.

Protected Time

It proved impossible to secure sufficient time for staff to participate fully in the project. Time was not protected for the meetings on the ward. For example in one 10-minute meeting, the matron was called away three times. The ward meetings were not consistently held or well attended, again indicative of the time pressures and workloads in the practice setting. Faced with extensive and complex patient care needs, staff had little or no opportunity to address their own needs for support in the context of a normal working day.

The Importance of Emotional Support

The need to care for each other in order to provide compassionate care for patients was recognised, but it was not addressed purposefully. Staff maintained that they 'did look out for each other', although a number of accounts of very stressful events, with no support being offered at the time or later on, were shared by staff. For example one nurse watched a distressing death, cleared up the blood, dealt with the relatives and left the ward without anyone asking her if she was all right. She described sitting in a bath with a glass of wine as an (ineffective) attempt to replenish her emotional resilience so as to be ready for her shift the next day.

Ability to Make the Changes

On the training days, staff identified changes that could be made. One was to structure the beginning and end of shifts for a handover based on the Samaritans' debriefing model. Part of the normal nursing handover, where relevant patient information is passed on to the group of staff coming on duty, was to be set aside for staff to trial the debriefing model – that is, enabling staff to discuss the following questions: what issues have you faced today which have upset or disturbed you, and how do you feel now? However, in the event, implementing even this seemingly minor change proved to be too difficult.

Although this is disappointing, it demonstrates the challenges involved in addressing this area of practice, and by using an action research methodology, the lessons learned can be built into the next iteration. This led to the following recommendations for future studies:

> Any initiatives to improve staff support and the provision of compassionate care need to be "owned" by the organisation.

➢ There needs to be visible and sustained senior management support, commitment from and practical support for the ward leader, and willingness of the whole team.

➢ There is no single solution, approaches need to be developed for each team in context.

➢ Approaches such as this are only one element in bringing about cultural change and will not work in isolation.

➢ More research is needed in this area to develop an evidence base for effective interventions (Sawbridge and Hewison, 2014: 9–10).

In terms of the final recommendation, a second action research project[1] is in progress in two different Trusts to explore how teams can best manage staff support.

Conclusion

Recognising that emotional labour is a role requirement for nursing is crucial if compassionate care is to be provided for patients. The ability of individuals to sustain the delivery of compassionate care is affected by the support they receive and has a direct impact on levels of compassion shown to patients by staff (Menzies, 1960; Maben, 2012; Smith, 2012). This needs to be understood and addressed in management practice. However, there is little evidence to suggest that this is the case. Recognising emotional labour is not just a good thing to do for nurses; it is also an important part of caring for patients and therefore core business for all healthcare organisations.

As Jocelyn Cornwell argued in her King's Fund blog (2011):

> Staff don't need more blame and condemnation; they need active, sustained supervision and support. In the high-volume, high-pressure, complex environment of modern healthcare it is very difficult to remain sensitive and caring towards every single patient all of the time. We ask ourselves how it is possible that anyone, let alone a nurse, could ignore a dying man's request for water? What we should also ask is whether it is humanly possible for anyone to look after very sick, very frail, possibly incontinent, possibly confused patients without excellent induction, training, supervision and support.

It may seem counterintuitive to suggest that nurses need to be valued and supported when there is a public outcry to address poor practice and hold people to account. However, if we are serious about solving the current concerns, the evidence suggests that understanding and responding to the needs of emotional labourers may be the missing link.

Note

1. Funded by Health Education West Midlands.

References

Ball, J. E., T. Murrells, A. M. Rafferty et al. (2014) '"Care Left Undone" during Nursing Shifts: Associations with Workload and Perceived Quality of Care', *British Medical Journal Quality and Safety*, 23(2): 116–25.

Bolton, S. C. and C. Boyd (2003) 'Trolley Dolly or Skilled Emotion Manager? Moving on from Hochschild's Managed Heart', *Work, Employment and Society*, 17(2): 289–308.

Bone, D. (2002) 'Dilemmas of Emotion Work in Nursing under Market-driven Healthcare', *International Journal of Public Sector Management*, 15(2): 140–50.

Bowling, A. (2002) *Research Methods in Health – Investigating Health and Health Services*, 2nd edn (Buckingham: Open University Press).

Bridges, J., C. Nicholson, J. Maben, C. Pope, M. Flatley et al. (2012) 'Capacity to Care: Meta-ethnography of Acute Nurses' Experiences of the Nurse–Patient Relationship', *Journal of Advanced Nursing*, 69(4): 760–72.

Care Quality Commission (CQC) (2011) *Dignity and Nutrition Inspection Programme: National Overview*, www.cqc.org.uk/file/4909, accessed 9 March 2015.

Cole-King, A. and P. Gilbert (2011) 'Compassionate Care: The Theory and the Reality', *Journal of Holistic Healthcare*, 8(3): 29.

Cornwell, J. (2011) 'Care and Compassion in the NHS', www.kingsfund.org.uk/blog/2011/02/care-and-compassion-nhs-patient-experience, accessed 13 August 2014.

Francis, R. (2010) *Independent Inquiry into Care Provided by Mid Staffordshire January 2005 to March 2009*, www.gov.uk/government/publications/independent-inquiry-into-care-provided-by-mid-staffordshire-nhs-foundation-trust-january-2001-to-march-2009, accessed 9 March 2015.

Francis, R. (2013) *Report of the Mid Staffordshire NHS Foundation Trust Public Inquiry*. Vols. 1–3, www.midstaffspublicinquiry.com/report, accessed 20 February 2014.

Gray, B. and P. Smith (2009) 'Emotional Labour and the Clinical Settings of Nursing Care: The Perspectives of Nurses in East London', *Nurse Education in Practice*, 9(4): 253–61.

Guy, M. E., M. A. Newman and S. H. Mastracci (2008) *Emotional Labor – Putting the Service in Public Service* (London: M. E. Sharpe).

Hart, E. and M. Bond (1995) *Action Research for Health and Social Care* (Buckingham: Open University Press).

Hochschild, A. R. (1983) *The Managed Heart: Commercialization of Human Feeling* (Berkeley: University of California Press).

Iles, V. (2011) *Why Reforming the NHS Doesn't Work: The Importance of Understanding How Good People Offer Bad Care*, www.reallylearning.com/Free_Resources/Really_Managing_Healthcare/reforming.pdf, accessed 13 August 2014.

kcl.ac.uk, (2012) 'King's College London – Staff Wellbeing Impacts Patient Experience', www.kcl.ac.uk/nursing/newsevents/news/2012/Staff-wellbeing-impacts-patient-experience.aspx, accessed 20 February 2015.

Leiter, M. P. and C. Maslach (1988) 'The Impact of Interpersonal Environment on Burnout and Organizational Commitment', *Journal of Organizational Behavior*, 9(4): 297–308.

Maben, J., R. Peccei, M. Adams, G. Robert, A. Richardson, T. Murrells and E. Morrow (2012) 'Patients' Experiences of Care and the Influence of Staff Motivation, Affect and Wellbeing', final report, NIHR Service Delivery and Organisation Programme.

Marrin, M. (2009) 'Fallen Angels – The Nightmare Nurses Protected by Silence', *Sunday Times*, 30 August, www.thesundaytimes.co.uk/sto/news/Features/Focus/article183320.ece, accessed 9 March 2015.

Maslach, C. (2003) *Burnout: The Cost of Caring* (Los Altos, CA: Malor Books).

Mastracci, S. E., M. E. Guy and M. A. Newman (2012) *Emotional Labor and Crisis Response – Working on the Razor's Edge* (London: M.E. Sharpe).

Melley, J. (2014) 'More Paramedics Quitting NHS Jobs', www.bbc.co.uk/news/uk-29542387, accessed 9 March 2015.

Menzies, I. E. P. (1960) 'A Case-Study in the Functioning of Social Systems as a Defence against Anxiety: A Report on a Study of the Nursing Service of a General Hospital', *Human Relations*, 13(2): 95–121.

NHS Alliance (2014) 'Think Big, Act Now: Creating a Community of Care', www.nhsalliance.org/wp-content/uploads/2014/10/THINK-BIGACT-NOW-FINAL-1.pdf, accessed 9 March 2015.

NHS Employers, Health, Safety and Wellbeing Partnership Group (2013) 'Workplace Health and Safety Standards', www.nhsemployers.org/~/media/Employers/Publications/workplace-health-safety-standards.pdf, accessed 9 March 2015.

Odone, C. (2011) 'Sulky, Lazy and Patronising: Finally, We Admit the Existence of the Bad Nurse, the NHS's Dirty Little Secret', *Daily Telegraph*, 12 April, http://blogs.telegraph.co.uk/news/cristinaodone/100083415/sulky-lazy-and-patronising-finally-we-admit-the-existence-of-the-bad-nurse-the-nhss-dirty-little-secret/, accessed 9 March 2015.

Osborne, S. (2014) 'How Can Nurses Show Compassion in 7.5 Minutes an Hour?', www.safestaffing.org.uk/the-alliance/how-can-nurses-show-compassion-in-7-5-minutes-an-hour/, accessed 10 March 2015.

Peate, I. (2014) 'Compassion Fatigue: The Toll of Emotional Labour', *British Journal of Nursing*, 23(5): 251.

The Press Association (2015) 'Nurses and Healthcare Staff Working Four Hours Unpaid Every Week', www.careappointments.co.uk/care-news/england/

item/36464-nurses-healthcare-staff-working-4-hours-unpaid-every-week, accessed 9 March 2015.

Queen's Nursing Institute (2014) '2020 Vision 5 Years on. Reassessing the Future of District Nursing', www.qni.org.uk/docs/2020_Vision_Five_Years_On_Web1.pdf, accessed 9 March 2015.

Rowland, E. J. (2014) *Emotional Geographies of Care Work in the NHS*. PhD thesis, Royal Holloway University of London, https://kclpure.kcl.ac.uk/portal/en/publications/emotional-geographies-of-care-work-in-the-nhs per cent28e8d893c2-9a35-42e9-ac62-9e550f0a21c0 per cent29.html, accessed 9 March 2015.

Royal College of Nursing (RCN) (2013a) 'RCN Employment Survey', www.rcn.org.uk/__data/assets/pdf_file/0005/541292/Employment_Survey_2013_004_503_FINAL_100214.pdf, accessed 9 March 2015.

Royal College of Nursing (RCN) (2013b) *Beyond Breaking Point? A Survey Report of RCN Members on Health, Well-Being and Stress*, www.rcn.org.uk/__data/assets/pdf_file/0005/541778/004448.pdf, accessed 9 March 2015.

Sawbridge, Y. and A. Hewison (2011) 'Time to Care: Responding to Concerns about Poor Nursing Care', www.birmingham.ac.uk/Documents/college-social-sciences/social-policy/HSMC/publications/PolicyPapers/policy-paper-twelve-time-to-care.pdf, accessed 13 August 2014.

Sawbridge, Y. and A. Hewison (2014) 'Time to Care? Report of an Action Research Project to Examine the Feasibility of Introducing the Samaritans' Volunteer Support System in Acute NHS Hospital Wards', www.birmingham.ac.uk/Documents/college-social-sciences/social-policy/HSMC/publications/2014/Time-To-Care-FINAL-March-2014.pdf, accessed 13 August 2014.

Smith, P. (1992) *The Emotional Labour of Nursing* (Basingstoke: Macmillan Education).

Smith, P. (2012) *The Emotional Labour of Nursing Revisited. Can Nurses Still Care?*, 2nd edn (Basingstoke: Palgrave Macmillan).

Turner, B. S. (1987) *Medical Power and Social Knowledge* (London: Sage).

Waddington, K. and C. Fletcher (2005) 'Gossip and Emotion in Nursing and Health-care Organizations', *Journal of Health Organization and Management*, 19(4/5): 378–94.

Youngson, R. A. (2012) *Time to Care: How to Love Your Patients and Your Job* (Raglan, New Zealand: Rebelheart).

9

Managing for Compassion

Valerie Iles

Introduction

We sometimes forget that managing people and organisations is primarily a human-to-human activity and that we can manage in ways that encourage and foster compassion among those humans or in ways that limit it.

Humans are complex, the result of millennia of evolution, and although we have the capacity for a wide range of behaviours, those we adopt are often not consciously chosen, but are instinctive responses to our perception of the situations we face. Thus to understand how people behave in ways that are less compassionate than we would like, we need to explore both their context and our human instincts.

In this chapter, I identify some of the historical, technological, sociological, political and economic factors that individually and cumulatively determine the situations which healthcare workers face daily.

We will see how they lead to a diminution of compassion in the day-to-day engagement between healthcare professionals (HCPs) and patients, between managers and HCPs and between commissioners and providers.

We also explore how we can help people be more emotionally 'resource-full', so they are able to choose more compassionate responses to the situations they face.

The discussion developed in this chapter draws on my experience of working with, and learning from, health professionals and managers over many years. It also summarises arguments and lines of inquiry I have explored in more detail elsewhere (Iles, 2011). The aim here is to illustrate the impact that social and organisational forces can have on compassion. In view of this, the approach taken is different to that taken in earlier chapters. The aim of this chapter is to synthesise a broad range of perspectives and experience to provide what I hope will be useful insights on the challenges facing all those concerned with delivering compassionate care. My intention is to be thought-provoking and to encourage you to reflect on your practice. With this in mind, references are used sparingly, as the points I make are grounded in a melding of experience, extensive reading and continuous reflection. I hope it helps you to consider your practice in a wider context.

Significant Factors Influencing Today's Healthcare: Environment

Factor 1: Technological Advances and Changing Demography

Over the last 150 years, health and healthcare have been transformed by public health measures (such as clean water, sewage systems, and better housing and heating) and advances in healthcare technologies (the most significant of all being the introduction of antibiotics, but also other advances in pharmaceuticals and medical devices) (Baggott, 2004). As a result, in Western economies there has been an increase in longevity across populations as a whole that is little short of amazing. This, combined with advances in birth control, has profoundly changed the demography of our societies (WHO, 2011).

There are now more fit, active older people within our communities, as well as more people with multiple morbidities who are supported by complex regimens of pharmaceutical and medical interventions, and more frail people over the age of 85 years. At the same time, there are comparatively fewer children and young people (WHO, 2011).

This has led some observers to wonder whether these changes have outpaced the ability of society to accommodate such dramatic demographic shifts. For example Steve Onyett drew on a tradition of 'council' (Transform, 2010) to suggest we have not developed community rituals (that in many societies mark the move from one role in society to another as members grow from childhood to adulthood) that fit these new life stages. Without these, our society has no way of harnessing the wisdom that such traditions foster. Instead, this time period has witnessed unprecedented geographic mobility and a collapse in traditional organised religion. So not only are there no community rituals accommodating our increased longevity, but there are also fewer communities.

Similarly Tim Dartington (2010) describes these developments as the 'adolescentisation of society': 'Society has become acculturated to what we may recognise as adolescent behaviour.' This is, he suggests, characterised by desperate but temporary attachments, fierce competitiveness, preoccupation with status and self-absorbed people confusing high ideals and selfish acts. It is a society, he observes, in which morality is built on fairness, in which the ambition is to get more and more in order to have one's 'fair share'.

These descriptions are vivid and arresting but we probably recognise them as only partial truths: as the society portrayed in our media but exhibited in *part* rather than in *all* of our lives. Nevertheless, it contributes to the culture in which caregivers are seeking to offer compassionate care to care seekers. It is a culture in which all are experiencing pressures towards adolescentisation, without contrasting support for the development of wisdom and maturity. It is not surprising, then, if our older citizens do not routinely adopt the more compliant and self-sacrificing behaviours of their predecessors, nor that professionals can derive more satisfaction from their competence, status and salary than from their relationships with their community.

Recognising these dynamics may allow us to consider ways of fostering maturity and wisdom and to change the context in which care is sought and offered.

Factor 2: The Digital Revolution

Although the term *digital revolution* is in common use (Peck and Phillips, 2008), not many of us pause to consider quite how revolutionary our ability to collect, store, move, compare and mine data has become. It has brought about huge changes in our leisure and entertainment options (although not without concomitant disbenefits in terms of reduced physical activity and concentration!). It has also led to major shifts in employment patterns as we all become our own (sometimes frustrated!) physician assistants, librarians, travel agents, bank clerks, data managers and so on.

It has also led to even more fundamental changes in the way we make judgements about the performance of individuals and organisations, and hence in our way of seeing the world. Consider, for example, the way the digital revolution has opened up many aspects of professional decision-making to external scrutiny. The use of the computer to record key points from client or clinician conversations and the treatments prescribed therein has created a means to compare and monitor the performance of individual clinicians, teams and organisations as a whole. Performance, in this sense, is judged against particular observable and measurable criteria, for example whether blood pressure has been checked or statins prescribed.

Similarly, when decisions are made about operational issues or about organisational strategy, discussions are recorded and minutes kept. Looking these up to trace the pathway of the decisions and the factors taken into account would, until recently, have required tenacity, time, physical access to records and some understanding of the issues involved. Now many such records are available almost instantly to anyone with access to the Internet.

Our ability to measure relative performance in this way, or to trace the path of a decision-making process, has led to increasing calls for the setting of performance objectives, for targets, for transparency and for more information about performance to be made available so that this can inform choice and also inform decisions about litigation. These calls have resulted in many countries introducing freedom of information legislation (e.g. UK Government, 2000; US Government, n.d.).

All of this sounds positive or, at worst, neutral in effect. It assumes that observing an individual, team or organisation simply gives us information about what they are doing and how. However, the act of observation affects the process being observed (Gillespie, 1991), and the nature of the data collected digitally changes it quite profoundly, as we shall see in the next section.

Factor 3: A Culture of Audit

Audit involves the examination of a process or an outcome against a defined standard and has led to some positive results: substandard practice can be identified and addressed, and there has been a standardisation of care in which unacceptable variation in outcomes is much reduced and good practice is more quickly shared. However, not all kinds of information are amenable to being collected or codified, and the digital revolution has, to date, succeeded in using (and therefore privileging) only the data that can. The resulting audit culture (Strathern, 2000) thus measures only some of the things we may deem to be important, and there are significant negative consequences of this.

> ➤ *A decreasing ability to handle uncertainty and tolerate ambiguity.* Audits, data comparisons and league tables fuel an illusion that we can *know*, that we can be *certain* about things for which that simply isn't the case. For example much is made of performance league tables, to aid our ability to decide about things like the education of our children. Surely this is an area for thoughtful, investigative judgement rather than a spurious certainty that our children will fare better at a school with a higher placing. Not only does this mislead, but it diminishes our skills in making those judgements.

> ➤ *A reduction in creativity.* When performance is measured against objectives, these objectives are required to be specified in advance. Although this is often a valuable discipline, there are many settings where the precise nature of the endeavour will not be known in advance, and there will be an *element* of emergent creativity in very many more.

Thus even where these objectives are set by the people closest to the activity, this very act of specifying them prevents any creativity or innovation being included when performance is monitored and published. Creativity and innovation are thus given lower priority than performing in accordance with the predefined agreements.

➢ When thinking ahead about what we will achieve over the next year (or even sometimes the next shift) we cannot know what new opportunities may arise, what problems, or what new insights we may gain. All of these may change our outlook and what it is we care about achieving, but if we have specified tight objectives in advance we do not allow ourselves to be creative in the ways in which we achieve what it is we really care about.

➢ *The only aspects that matter are those that can be codified.* Only activities that *can* be measured *are* measured – so this privileges the use of explicit knowledge over tacit knowledge, and activity at the expense of thinking. It is these measurable 'facts' and activities that are then the basis of 'performance' as made public. In the area of professional decision-making, judgement and 'practical wisdom' are an essential feature, and the wisdom drawn upon to inform an act is as important as the act itself but is not (and cannot be) captured. Thus 'hyperactivity and discourse are privileged over wisdom and silence'.

➢ *We don't measure what is happening, only how we are managing what is happening.* As a result of the points discussed above, there are difficulties in capturing the nature of 'first-order activities' (in healthcare these first-order activities are the interactions between professionals and patients and/or the clinical outcomes of these), and thus it is not these that are monitored, but second-order processes. These second-order processes are supposed to ensure delivery of the essential first-order activity and include a range of governance activities and performance targets. However, the link between these proxy indicators and the outcomes we seek is often not sound, and we divert resources away from what is important to what is measured. For example when the Labour Government wanted to improve the quality of service within the NHS, it chose to set performance targets including specifying that patients should wait no longer than four hours in A&E before being admitted to hospital or discharged and that patients must be treated within 18 weeks once referred to a hospital by their general practitioner.

➢ These could have been used as prompts to reflect on how to offer considerate compassionate care to all and in the process meet these targets. Instead, they became the entire focus of attention, and as a result many other aspects of patient care suffered. For example some patients were discharged in the middle of the night without any prior notice to free up beds for people from A&E to be admitted (see e.g. www.nhs. uk/news/2012/04april/Pages/nhs-hospital-discharge-times-examined. aspx).

➤ *Litigation increases and the lowest-risk option is privileged.* As more information becomes available (although not necessarily complete information – only that which is codified and stored), and as the understanding of the processes of professional decision-making and action becomes distorted (as a consequence of the points made above), so litigation increases. This in turn changes decision priorities, so that the lowest-risk option is often given automatic priority, even where there are sound arguments for others. After all, if it were not and the worst happened, those who took the decision would be pilloried and sued. This in turn leads to a preoccupation with risk, the development of risk registers and requirements to 'manage' risk (Beck, 1992), which all misunderstands the multifaceted *nature* of risk and its different meaning to different people. In fact, meaning is something the audit culture ignores (see for example www. scotland.gov.uk/Resource/Doc/194419/0052192.pdf). It is important to emphasise this changed attitude to risk. Not only does it become the predominant factor in every decision, risk is now something to be assessed and managed rather than taken. Furthermore, only the elements that are codifiable can be recorded, and those which cannot are not recognised. As a result, risk can become the acid bath that corrodes truth (Beck, 1992).

➤ *Policymakers set targets: local leaders game the system.* It becomes tempting for policymakers to respond to public dissatisfaction with a service by setting targets for particular aspects of it. These targets relate to easily measurable aspects that do not encompass the whole. The ways in which they can be met can be divided into those with integrity and those without – the latter being easier and quicker than the former. In other words, targets can be met as a result of improvements to the system, getting everyone involved to reflect on how things could be done differently and better. Or they can be met by focusing solely on the target at the expense of system.

➤ So as performance is measured only against these targets and not against the service as a whole, it is almost inevitable that those held 'personally accountable' for delivering targets find ways of meeting the targets that do not improve (or even worsen) the service, for example the ambulance service meeting the eight-minute response time to attend a patient who has a suspected stroke in his own home, by sending a paramedic on a motorcycle. The eight-minute target is met; however, what the patient needs is an ambulance to get them to hospital as soon as possible. In this way, the target is met, yet the care provided is not what the patient needs.

Factor 4: A Change in the Nature of Politics

For centuries, politics was essentially about the reconciling of different interests. It was not always enacted fairly or wisely, and democracy is a fairly late comer onto the scene, but in the memory of many the role of Government involved considering the well-being of citizens, encouraging and supporting commercial activity and balancing that with the need for a flourishing society egalitarian enough for the welfare of its citizens and the orderliness of Government, while also incentivising those with talent to use it for the benefit of society as well as themselves.

In the last 30–40 years, that has changed. At both a local and global level, the market is deemed to be the best way of allocating resources, and this changes the role of Government to that of ensuring that markets are in place and are functioning competitively. This involves setting the frameworks within which businesses compete and policing them to ensure they do so, with the aim of offering customers the most suitable products at the lowest prices. Where (as in health, social services, education and utilities) pure markets would fail, quasi-markets have been introduced, which means that instead of all the budget being spent on service delivery and its direct management, significant resources are used to commission services by specifying the service needed and offering different organisations the right to tender for contracts to offer that service.

It is important to note that there are logical arguments in support of this agenda (commonly known as a 'neoliberal' set of political policies based on a modified form of liberalism tending to favour free-market capitalism) just as there are against it. So the people holding these different views can share the same values (such as wanting the best healthcare for a population) but see different ways of achieving it.

It is also worth noting that one of the ways in which this change in role has been achieved (and is constantly being cemented) has been the denigration of the probity and motives of politicians.

The digital revolution has enabled a new form of journalism that hasn't favoured our political leaders. It is easy to make someone look foolish, indecisive or duplicitous when actually the person is being thoughtful, well intentioned and honest. In the course of exploring an issue, politicians may change their mind as they become more familiar with the complexities involved. So it is all too easy for the media to juxtapose clips of politicians espousing current and previous views and require them to undertake jousts with combative interviewers whose interest is more in reputation and audience figures than in effective democracy.

Sadly, this prevents policymakers from engaging in real discussion, real exploration, and real engagement with people who have first-hand experience of the impact of policy, so policy is informed less by experience, wisdom and valid experience, than by logic.

Factor 5: Managerialism

Another factor in this mix, arising from and contributing to the factors already mentioned, has been the development of a new style of management.

When organisations were small, management could consist largely of conversations. Shop floor workers could talk with their supervisors, who talked with department heads, who talked to the management team. In the latter half of the twentieth century, organisations grew larger (Watson, 2008). This occurred for many reasons, including technological advances, competitive markets leading to mergers and acquisitions, the development of IT systems that could monitor production and performance, and so on. As they became larger, organisations also became more similar, and skills in running a large organisation became seen as more relevant than experience in a particular industry or service, when appointing management teams.

This growing belief that management required a knowledge base of its own, armed with which managers could manage anything, anywhere, accompanied the rise of business schools. The analytical methods taught have led to generations of business school graduates now forming a management cadre that:

> has more faith in logic and very particular kinds of evidence than in wider forms of experience and judgement (i.e. explicit knowledge rather than tacit);

> relies on data dashboards and performance incentives rather than on relationships between managers and their staff; and

> prefers formal strategies based on analytics over an ability to respond sensitively to changes in circumstance (analysing situations as complicated rather than complex).

However, such approaches are of limited use when addressing 'puzzles' rather than 'problems or messes' (Ackoff, 1974).

Relations between management and professionals have suffered particularly badly in this process, as the essence of professionalism (and what distinguishes a professional from an expert technician) is the ability to bring experience and judgement to a situation – what, in complexity theory, is known as 'muddling through elegantly' (Hunter, 2001; Kernick, 2002) – whereas managerialism prefers standardised protocols. Of course there is a need for both, but in many settings relations have soured to the point that it can be difficult for this to be remembered.

Influences on Our Instinctive Responses

Underlying and exacerbating the factors discussed thus far, and a characteristic of our very existence, is our natural anxiety – our constant instinctive concern about anything that may cause us harm.

It is our anxiety that fuels our desire for certainty and for rankings of the performance of services on which we depend. It fuels our desire to have data evidence of the performance of people we are managing, rather than rely on our perceptions in response to conversations and other interactions with them. It also fuels our preference for logical explanations and prescriptions rather than trusting our experience and experience-informed intuitions.

Ironically too, our increasing longevity appears to have made us more rather than less anxious, less prepared to accept our fate and more concerned to influence it.

So we have all instinctively contributed to the factors described above and continue to do so, with both positive and negative results. Our anxiety, then, is both cause and result of the other factors and an important part of the context of care.

How Is This Affecting Care?

In the type of environment described above, compassion has to compete for attention with so many other concerns that consequently we cannot be surprised if it is not always paramount.

More than that: there is a danger that this context is leading to a change in the nature of care. A change in which patients are no longer cared *about* (I care about what happens to you and about how the quality of our interaction can help you, and I will make sure you get the best treatment for you, within the resources available) but cared *for* (you have condition X, for which the best, evidence-based, most cost-effective treatment is Y. I will make sure you get Y).

Increasingly, caregivers are required to offer care that is a set of auditable transactions between patients and professionals, with professionals becoming essentially a unit of production. Although these auditable transactions are important and necessary, often both care-seeker and care-giver want more from their interaction: they want a covenant of care in which they relate as people, and not only as fulfilment of a contract (Iles, 2011).

Table 9.1 illustrates the difference between these two ways of considering care. In the left-hand column, care is a set of auditable transactions in

Table 9.1 Transactional Care and Covenantal Care

Transactional Care	Covenantal Care
Healthcare as a set of auditable transactions in the market economy – patient as consumer, professional as provider	*Healthcare with elements of the gift economy. Care that results from a relationship, a covenant, between caregiver and receiver*
Patient is cared for.	Patient is cared about as well as for.
Professionals are seen as givers (or suppliers) of services.	Professionals recognise that in their encounters with patients they give *and* receive.
Focus is on calculation and counting – this can be seen as objective.	Focus is on thoughtful, purposeful judgement – this is necessarily subjective but incorporates objective measures and evidence.
There are predetermined protocols.	Emergent creativity which can include the use of protocols.
Discourse and hyperactivity set the model.	Wisdom and silence are valued in addition to discourse and action.
Explicit knowledge is held in high regard.	Both tacit knowledge and explicit knowledge are seen as important.
Reflection is based on facts and figures.	Reflection centres on feelings and ethics as well.
Focus is on dealing with the presenting problem.	The meaning of the encounter – for both parties – is kept in mind while addressing the presenting problem.
Competence is what is called for on the part of the professional.	The humanity of the professional is also called upon.
Individuals have a relationship with the state and with the market.	Individuals have a relationship with the community and with wider society.
Good policy ideas *must* degenerate as they are translated at every level of the system into a series of measurable, performance manageable actions and objectives. The focus here is on being able to demonstrate the policy has been implemented.	Policy ideas can stay rich and be added to creatively so that solutions are responsive, humane, practical, flexible and adaptable. Here the focus is on solving problems.

a market or quasi-market. In the right-hand column, these auditable transactions are achieved but offered in ways that involve elements of a gift economy as well. The key differences between a market and gift economy are listed in Table 9.2.

Table 9.2 The Differences between a Market Economy and a Gift Economy[1]

In a Market Economy	In a Gift Economy
Status is gained according to what we acquire (which can be material goods or things like power).	Status is gained according to what we give away.
We talk of value. Value can usually be expressed in monetary terms and allows us to compare and trade things that are completely unlike each other.	We talk of worth. The worth of an object has nothing to do with its monetary value. The worth of a painting is to do with the labour (see below) of the artist and the reaction of the viewer.
We describe our efforts as work: we can measure the skills we deploy and energy we put in for a given time period.	We describe our efforts as labour: we give something of ourselves; what we do includes some essence of ourselves and cannot be measured in the quantitative terms favoured by contemporary management.

[1] See Lewis Hyde (2007) *The Gift: How the Creative Spirit Transforms the World* (London: Canongate).

The elements of 'transactional care' are all necessary, and on many occasions they will be sufficient, but there will be occasions when something more like a relationship will also be important (for both parties). Another way of describing this is as a covenant of care. Unfortunately, exchanges in the gift economy do not lend themselves to being codified and captured, so do not receive the senior organisational attention and priority they warrant.

The pressure to perform and record the activities in the left-hand column, with little reference to those of the right, can provoke resistance from clinicians, and as attention to both columns is needed, organisational managers must take sufficient interest in the right if clinicians are to do the same for the left.

It can be argued that the requirements listed in the right-hand column require additional time, whereas others (myself included) suggest that feeling emotionally resource-full (calm, confident and unpressured) is more important.

Practical Steps We Can Take

Given the range of factors contributing to the complex situation in which compassion can be lost, it is tempting to feel there is nothing that we, as individuals or small groups, can do. But it is our anxiety that is at the root of this situation, and our compliance that endorses it. If we can change our own responses, we can increase the chance of more compassionate care becoming the norm.

So what can we do to help increase the levels of compassion in our organisations?

Emotional Resourcing

If we are to work in a covenant of care, we need to equip ourselves emotionally and see this as important in ensuring that we have all the kit and other resources we may need to provide physical care.

We all have three major emotional systems, which can be thought of as the fight/flight system; the incentive/resource-seeking system; and the soothing/contentment system (Gilbert, 2009), which need to be kept in balance if we are to flourish, and especially if we are to be compassionate. If we keep this in mind we can find ways of providing that balance for ourselves, and those around us. We can even design some of our routine organisational processes to support that balance.

Typically, though, our routine systems are focused on minimising risk and primarily activate our fight-or-flight system. Think of ward handovers for instance, in which one shift hands over to the next by highlighting the risks to be averted and avoided. In a little more time, we could choose to activate the soothing/connecting system by celebrating things that have gone well in the last shift, involve our incentive/resource-seeking system by setting some positive ambitions for the next shift and make our mention of risk a part of an endeavour that is altogether more energising and rewarding. On occasion, we will need to mourn too, but mourn rather than blame and hide.

Responding Mindfully

As the fundamental cause of the factors described above is our anxious, unhelpful, instinctive response to situations, perhaps the most important thing we can do is to become more aware of our patterns of reacting – to become more mindful, more aware of our responses as they arise, to recognise them and give ourselves the choice of whether to accede or to substitute a different, more considered response.

There are many programmes of mindfulness and meditation that focus on exactly this, and even a brief introduction to the principles – especially if supported with some short, simple practices that can be fitted into odd moments during a day – can be transformative.

We can, for example, learn to identify and consider healthy responses to anxiety instead of our instinctive unhealthy (mindless) ones. The differences between them are listed in Table 9.3.

Table 9.3 Healthy and Unhealthy Responses to Anxiety[2]

Healthy Responses to Anxiety	Unhealthy Responses to Anxiety
Recognising it and bringing it into awareness	Criticising or blaming others This is such a common response that we can begin to recognise that whenever we find ourselves criticising or blaming another, we are responding unhealthily to an anxiety, and can use this to bring our anxiety into awareness.
Reflecting on it and identifying the source of it What is the fear of our own behind it, e.g.: ➢ that we do not have the skills and may cause harm or discomfort to another or to our own reputation? ➢ that we do not want to invest time in this when there are other things we dearly long to do? ➢ that we do not know how others will react, or fear they will react emotionally, and do not know how we will handle that?	Rushing into action or actions that may not be the most valuable (e.g. looking instantly for a suitable protocol for care before really understanding the issues, concerns and expectations of the patient) This ready action relieves us of the anxiety.
Seeking support if we need it	Not seeking support when it is needed
Reminding ourselves of our sense of purpose: what is it we care deeply about achieving in our work? What kind of energy do we want to live from?	Finding something that needs doing that can take us away from the source of the anxiety Stock takes and other forms of counting, such as looking at the patient's chart, are common. Or returning to our computer screen, where we are likely to find requests and deadlines for reports, etc., imposed by other people (to which we may feel we must respond and who we can then blame).

Thinking carefully about the needs and wishes of the other	
Thinking clearly about these various concerns and interests (our own and those of the other) so that we are able to make a free choice about how to respond	
That response may be a decision to embark on a course of 'aware altruism', the taking on of a difficult or distasteful task because of our concern for others and our preparedness to put their needs ahead of our own preferences.	
It may result in a meaningful dialogue with the other, without knowing what the outcome of the conversation will be and tolerating that uncertainty.	
Or it may involve seeking support from someone more skilled in a particular procedure.	

[2] This is described in more detail in Iles (2011).

We can learn too to tolerate situations of ambiguity and uncertainty, recognising our natural distaste for these and choosing to stay with them instead of instinctively getting rid of them by jumping to judgement or conclusion.

By becoming more familiar with our instinctive mental patterns, we empower ourselves to choose differently, and in doing so to build our ability to choose to be compassionate even when to be so is difficult, distasteful or back-breaking.

Understanding Complexity

Complex situations are just that. They are what systems theorist Russell Ackoff (1974) termed 'messes'. They are not 'puzzles' (where there is a right answer) or 'problems' (where there is no right answer, but better and worse approaches). They are complex dynamic systems of many interacting problems and puzzles in which the only effective way forward is to 'muddle through elegantly'. Such muddling through is something that professional judgement is all about; it is what Aristotle (whose other work was considered in Chapter 2) called practical wisdom. Analyses and data can help inform decisions, but because they cannot represent the full complexity, they can never yield answers.

The implications of this are profound and unsettling for those who like life to be ordered and predictable, with effects directly resulting logically from particular causes.

It means, for example, that it is often inappropriate or even wrong to ascribe blame to individuals or groups when the outcome of a complex situation is painful or unpleasant. To blame someone who was 'muddling through' as elegantly as they (or anyone else) could, when a way forward was not clear and where the outcome depended on all sorts of chances and interactions that were beyond the control or even sight of that person, is an example of 'spurious retrospective coherence' (Iles, 2014). To look back and say that A led to B, and that therefore the person doing A was to blame, ignores the fact that A often doesn't lead to B; indeed, it only does if G takes place, and that only happens if both L and P do happen and Z doesn't, and if S and X interact to produce F, which they sometimes do and sometimes don't … for example:

It's often better to turn left at these traffic lights, so today, as we are keen not to be late, I decide to do that. How sure can we be that we will get to our appointment on time? Is that a puzzle, a problem or a mess? Let's see.

How long it takes us will depend on whether the schools are on holiday. Today they are, so that should make it easier for us. But our journey time also depends on whether there is a hold-up on the M25 – two miles away – and that depends on whether there has been an accident on the M1, 10 miles away. Normally, the M1 is clear at this time, but in school holidays it can bunch up and be more unpredictable.

It will also depend on what time of day it is, and whether this is one of the three days a week that the delivery van calls at the pharmacy on the high road, where it sometimes causes a blockage, especially if the supermarket van is unloading at the same time. And sometimes there are exceptional circumstances (a very high volume of additional prescriptions for flu jabs perhaps) when an extra delivery will be scheduled. Shortage of staff at your workplace is the reason we have to be on time today, and I'm not feeling at my best and am slightly worried I'm suffering the first flu symptoms, so I'm not thinking as clearly as usual. You have already spotted that.

So if we turn left and get stuck in traffic and you are late – whose fault is that? I took the critical decision that turned out to be wrong – this time, in these particular circumstances, which are unlikely to be exactly replicated on any other day. Looking back afterwards, we can see that it was the wrong decision, but at the time I took it, that simply wasn't clear. I was making a decision I've made before that has often worked before. To blame me would be an example of spurious retrospective coherence.

When something goes wrong we need to seek to understand not to blame.

It also means that we cannot expect to progress to a defined future state from our current messy one by producing a plan and sticking to it, no matter how much analysis has been done to support the production of the plan. So when we decide that a current situation is causing us problems, the answer is not to logically analyse data and formulate a plan and then stringently project-manage its implementation with the aim of achieving a neatly defined future state.

After all, the future is bound to be messy too – the present always is whenever it takes place. We will always be in a situation in which there are lots of things going well and badly and helpfully and unhelpfully. That is called life. There is a traditional Sufi saying that life consists of ten thousand joys and ten thousand sorrows, and perhaps it is time we revisited the wisdom of that instead of believing that we can magically wish away the sorrows.

We would be much better advised to try to understand our current 'mess', its dynamics, and help others to understand it along with us. Once we have all done that and can all see the current or imminent problems that are inherent in it, then we can all take the individual actions that will cumulatively result in change. So if we are to take complexity seriously, we need to develop leaders who can help people to explore and understand complex dynamics, encourage a sense of personal agency so that we all feel we can do something that will make a difference (indeed that everything we do has an effect) and sometimes provide a sense of urgency to generate the energy we need to think creatively about the changes we can make.

Managing People, Not Performance

We are all complex mixtures of virtues and vices – for example of altruism and endeavour plus self-righteous complacency. We can all be encouraged to spend more time in our caring, connected, contributing self and less in our self-absorbed, greedy one by spending time with people who support us when we are behaving well and challenge us (gracefully but effectively) when we are not. For us to be influenced by those people, they need to know us and have confidence in us as a result of that knowledge; we need to trust that they understand us and have our interests at heart. We also need to be sure that they are competent in their own roles and have the interests of the wider service in mind.

Whatever we call this, 'management' or 'clinical supervision' or 'leadership' (personally I have always called it *'real* management' [Iles, 2006], it takes place through conversations between people who know each other. It is very different from today's management in which dashboards of data about our performance are scrutinised at a distance by people we may never meet.

What we need is a covenant of care between caregivers and their managers that parallels that described above between caregivers and care seekers.

Valuing Expertise

There is a difference between technical experts and professionals. Technical expertise is always used in the same way. Professional expertise is deployed with judgement – it includes a lot of technical expertise, but that expertise can be used differently according to the circumstances in which it is needed. The judgement is vital and is not held by those without that professional expertise. Tasks can be delegated, but the judgement cannot. So replacing expensive staff with cheaper ones is sometimes a good use of resources and sometimes a false economy. The loss is felt by people whose carers are following protocols or algorithms and do not have the autonomy to make compassionate judgements about what care is needed. Indeed, this is what led to the growth of a community nursing organisation in the Netherlands called Buurtzorg (Laloux, 2014). Teams of 12 qualified nurses provide all the home care to their patients according to their needs, and have the freedom to use their professional judgements in a manner almost inconceivable in the UK.

At the same time as we are replacing nurses with care assistants, and doctors with nurses, we are dispensing with the services of medical secretaries and other support staff that have traditionally enabled clinicians to use their time to best effect. It is often the digital revolution that has allowed this, but we do need to look at the amount of time that is spent by professionals on activities that could be better and more cheaply done by support staff.

Instead of replacing expensive people with cheaper ones, we need to encourage our expensive staff to behave in ways that make us find them indispensible. We need to help our expensive people behave expensively. For example:

> We need people who hold high social status (such as many health-care professionals) to use their status wisely and well, and not unwittingly abuse it. So if we are discussing arrangements in an operating theatre, and a consultant surgeon gives considerable thought to the matter and makes a set of proposals that are based on his understanding of the evidence and on his clinical

experience, and he is clearly more concerned for the safety of patients than for his own convenience, then he is using his expensively acquired expertise well. He is behaving like an expensive person. Now imagine one of his colleagues is arguing about having a place in the car park so that he can drop his children at school on the way. That place would otherwise go to the community nursing team who, without parking arrangements, are being required to use public transport, and as a result are often late for appointments and causing distress to their patients. I suggest that the surgeon is not thinking of the best for patients; he is not drawing on his professional expertise, nor taking account of relevant evidence. So here he is not using his status appropriately. He is not behaving as an expensive person; he is simply fighting for his own convenience. We need to help people to distinguish between these behaviours, and that is what I mean by helping expensive people to behave expensively.

We need to give them the support they need so that they can focus on tasks and situations that need their expertise, and not waste their time on aspects that can be undertaken better and more cheaply by someone else. At the same time, we need to encourage them to take a wider interest in the total experience of their patients and indeed of all patients attending their hospital, and not only on the conditions in which they play their own part. If they took an interest in factors that affect that experience (such as patient administration systems for example, or nursing ratios on wards) and contributed constructively to discussions about how best to allocate resources, better decisions could be taken and could be implemented more smoothly.

Fighting Ideas and Not People

We are all battling to survive and thrive in a morass of forces and factors, and we develop different strategies to do so and different ideas about how things should be organised for the world to be a good place to live in.

As we do, we come across people with different ideas from our own, and it is all too easy for us to dislike these people rather than their ideas. That way lies huge danger (as we witness daily in news programmes on our television screens).

Where we see things that are of great value to society, then, we should indeed put energy into ensuring they remain if they are threatened. We are more likely to be successful if we find allies to work with and if we can make a case to the people who think differently to us that recognises their concerns and values are very similar to ours; it is just the strategies for delivering them that differ.

Personalising debates makes it almost impossible for the other party to hear what we are saying, makes us look childish and leads only to an increase in anger on all sides. Presenting and exploring opposing ideas is much more important, much more interesting and in everyone's interests. It requires us as readers and contributors to fora such as social media to resist the temptation to join a fight between personalities and stick to thoughtful responses to ideas.

Conclusion

If we are to influence the level of compassion on offer in society, including that of caregivers to care seekers in the NHS, we need to understand the factors that shape the context in which care is undertaken. These are multiple and interact in a complex system that we can (like Russell Ackoff, 1974) term a 'mess'.

When we appreciate this complexity, we can, instead of leaping to judgement and blame, and instead of prescribing new systems and punishments, choose to change our own responses to daily situations and in doing so change the world.

Useful Resources/Websites

http://hostleadership.com/steve-onyett-1961-2015/.

Xformedit, 'The Way of Council', Transform, 5 February 2010, http://transform. transformativechange.org/2010/02/the-way-of-council/.

T. Dartington, 'Managing Vulnerability: The Underlying Systems of the Dynamics of Care', The Tavistock Institute, June 2010, www.tavinstitute.org/ news/managing-vulnerability-the-underlying-dynamics-of-systems-of-care.

References

Ackoff, R. L. (1974) *Redesigning The Future: A Systems Approach to Societal Problems* (New York: Wiley).

Baggot, R. (2004) *Health and Healthcare in Britain*, 3rd edn (Basingstoke: Palgrave Macmillan).

Beck, U. (1992) *Risk Society – Towards a New Modernity* (London: Sage).

Dartington, T. (2010) 'Managing Vulnerability: The Underlying Dynamics of Systems of Care', The Tavistock Institute, June, www.tavinstitute.org/news/ managing-vulnerability-the-underlying-dynamics-of-systems-of-care.

Gilbert, P. (2009) *The Compassionate Mind* (London: Constable and Robinson).

Gillespie, G. (1991) *Manufacturing Knowledge, A History of the Hawthorne Experiments* (Cambridge: Cambridge University Press).

Hunter, D. J. (2001) 'Rationing Healthcare: The Appeal of Muddling through Elegantly', *Healthcare Papers*, 2(2): 31–7.

Hyde, L. (2007) *The Gift: How the Creative Spirit Transforms the World* (London: Canongate).

Iles, V. (2006) *Really Managing Healthcare* (Maidenhead: Open University Press).

Iles, V. (2011) 'Why Reforming the NHS Doesn't Work', www.reallylearning.com/Free_Resources/MakingStrategyWork/reforming.pdf, accessed 27 April 2016.

Iles, V. (2014) 'The Challenges of Leading Professionals', *The International Journal of Leadership in Public Services*, 10(1): 44–51.

Kernick, D. (ed.) (2002) *Getting Health Economics into Practice* (Oxford: Radcliffe Medical Press), www.onyett.org/about-steve-onyett, accessed 27 April 2016.

Peck, J. and R. Phillips (2008) *Citizen Renaissance* (digital book), www.citizenrenaissance.com/the-book/, accessed 4 March 2015.

Strathern, M. (ed.) (2000) *Audit Cultures: Anthropological Studies in Accountability, Ethics and the Academy* (Abingdon: Routledge).

Transform, 'The Way of Council', 5 February 2010, http://transform.transformativechange.org/2010/02/the-way-of-council/, accessed 27 April 2016.

UK Government (2000) Freedom of Information Act, www.legislation.gov.uk/ukpga/2000/36/contents, accessed 27 April 2016.

US Government (n.d.) http://foia.state.gov/, accessed 27 April 2016.

Watson, T. J. (2008) *Sociology, Work and Industry*, 5th edn (London: Routledge).

World Health Organization (WHO) (2011) 'Global Health and Aging', World Health Organization, www.nia.nih.gov/sites/default/files/global_health_and_aging.pdf, accessed 27 April 2016.

10

Restorative Supervision Implications for Nursing

Sonya Wallbank

Introduction

In this chapter, the model of Restorative Supervision, which has been used with a range of nursing and other professional care teams across the UK and internationally, will be discussed. The model (Wallbank, 2007) has been used with over 3500 individuals since 2007, and it is the learning from these sessions that this chapter reports.

We begin with a brief history of the model and its research roots, reflecting on other models of clinical supervision and how Restorative Supervision differs from them. The aim of the chapter is to support you in reflecting on the learning that has arisen about individual nurses from these sessions and how you might be able to use this information in your own professional development. In the main, nurses enter the profession because of their desire to care for others, and this in itself confers a greater vulnerability to the stresses and strains of the work. Managing and supporting yourself, alongside your own reaction to the work you are involved in, is often missed as an integral part of the emotional cost of the work you do. This chapter offers some insights into what increases a nurse's vulnerability and how you might like to think about your own techniques for maintaining and improving your resilience.

We then consider another important issue identified in the work on restorative supervision: how to work with people inside and outside your organisation. We reflect on the learning the sessions have generated about the wider organisation and how where you work can both mediate and exacerbate your capacity to think and care for the patients you are responsible for. Finally, the chapter aims to take you beyond your basic capacity to function as a nurse and support you to think about what you need to do in order to thrive in this environment.

Research Roots

The model of supervision and support was initially piloted with midwives, doctors and nurses in obstetric and gynaecology settings (Wallbank, 2007, 2010). The initial programme was developed in response to several years of research (Wallbank and Robertson, 2013) investigating the impact of stillbirth and miscarriage on professionals who cared for the families experiencing loss following these events.

The first study was designed to address the emotional impact on staff working in these areas, support them to build resilience and reduce their level of stress and burnout. The results showed restorative supervision increased compassion satisfaction (the pleasure derived from doing the job) as well as reducing burnout and stress by over 40 per cent (Wallbank, 2010). This was the first opportunity some professionals had experienced since qualifying to think about the emotional demands of their role, and the qualitative feedback described the positive impact on patient care of staff taking time to think.

Having an individual who is thinking clearly and can remain patient-centred at the bedside is critical for compassionate care. If nurses focus on the next thing in their head because they are overwhelmed by their work-load, they will appear distracted at best or disinterested at worst. Working in a stressed or overwhelmed state often means that our cognitive systems resort to 'thinking fast' (Kahneman, 2012). We operate on autopilot and become task-focused in an attempt to control the way we are feeling (Wallbank, 2007). The restorative sessions enable individuals to 'think slowly' (Kahneman, 2012), engage with patients on a more meaningful level and give of themselves emotionally without the anxiety that in doing so they risk burning themselves out. When reviewing the impact on patient care as reported by staff who have been through the programme, it appeared that the pleasure of providing care and support for patients was increased, and this meant they were more in tune with the patients' needs (DH, 2013).

Supporting staff to remain resilient in the care environment is not new. However, in the past, support has tended to be centred on more obvious psychologically demanding work such as oncology, terminal care and paediatrics. This was mainly due to the emotional demands of this work being recognised and appropriately supported. One of the main difficulties in any type of caring environment is that the day-to-day effort, the 'emotional labour' of caring work, is often not recognised (see Chapter 8).

The programme of restorative supervision developed from the initial studies has now been rolled out to over 3500 staff in hospitals, community settings and other care settings in the UK, Australia and Ireland. The results have been consistent, reducing burnout and stress and supporting participants to increase the pleasure they gain from their work and how they feel connected to their employment through compassion satisfaction (Wallbank, 2010, 2011, 2013a,b). Compassion satisfaction is the pleasure derived from being able to do your work well (Stamm, 2010). Experiencing positive feelings about work is highly protective against stress and burnout (Schaufeli and Bakker, 2004). In care settings, feeling that you have done a good enough job mediates the impact of the work on individual levels of resilience (Wallbank, 2007).

What Is the Approach?

Clinical supervision is a formal process of professional support that promotes self-assessment and analytical and reflexive skill-building. It can also support individual practitioners to develop knowledge and competence, assume responsibility for their own practice and enhance consumer protection and safety in complex situations (CIPD DH, 1993).

The main types of supervision are as follows:

> **Educational** – This type of supervision is directed towards the educational development of the practitioner and the fulfilment of potential. The supervisee is considered to have less experience and knowledge than the supervisor.

> **Administrative/Managerial** – This type of supervisory relationship is focused on the promotion and maintenance of quality standards, adherence to policies and good practice (Kadushin, 1992).

Proctor (1986) refers to the normative, formative and restorative aspects of supervision.

> **Normative** – Similar to the administrative or managerial function, the supervisor here accepts responsibility for the adherence of the supervisee to the professional and ethical standards of the organisation and job role.

> **Formative** – This is similar to the educational supervision outlined above. The supervisor provides feedback or direction for supervisees to help them become competent practitioners.

> **Restorative** – This type of supervision involves elements of psychological support including listening, supporting and challenging the supervisee to improve his or her capacity to cope, especially in managing difficult and stressful situations (Proctor, 1986).

A number of different models or methods are used for conducting clinical supervision, including group, multidisciplinary, network and individual supervision.

The restorative supervision model (Wallbank, 2007) is different to other approaches as it is concerned with the needs of staff members and how they interact with their caseload and workplace environment, rather than with the caseload itself. Supporting staff members to think more clearly and challenging their ways of working has a positive impact on their capacity to work with their caseload (DH, 2013; Wallbank and Woods, 2012). The programme starts with supporting individuals to reflect on their own capacity to think and what might be interfering with that. One thing that has been apparent from the beginning of this programme of work is that the scale and impact of the issues differ for each individual. At times it has been the cumulative effect of loss on the individual that has become difficult to bear. This was especially relevant in the work with nurses, doctors and midwives working with stillbirth and miscarriage. For example it was often not the most complex family with a challenging clinical picture that was difficult to manage, but the one that most touched them because of something that was said or done.

Some individuals are more resilient than others, and people react differently to each set of events. What touches individuals, and therefore what needs to be discussed and resolved, is unique to the individual's set of circumstances and his or her professional experiences. Restorative supervision allows time and space for these issues to be discussed, identifying the significance of particular events and ongoing workplace demands.

Participants being supervised in this way learn about the concepts, evidence and what will happen within the sessions before they begin supervision. This is crucial as it enables them to begin to prepare their own understanding of how to make best use of the time. Getting the supervisor and supervisee relationship right is a good start to any session, and preparing to think about this relationship is an excellent precursor to successful sessions.

In order to meet the needs of individuals, elements of the session must remain open so that the participants can utilise them as they see fit. There is no prescribed agenda, and the success of the session comes from the supervisor and the supervisee finding the best way to work together to generate productive learning from these experiences.

It is important to note that restorative supervision is not counselling, although the skills of active listening, reflecting and helping individuals to understand their situation are similar to those used by counsellors. The aim of restorative supervision is to use the discussion to support the supervisee. By holding a mirror up to ourselves, we understand why we have reacted in this way to this one situation when in other similar situations we have coped. Perhaps thinking about why this person or team is affecting how I am working, or why this manager and the way she or he behaves is undermining my confidence. Why has this patient got under my skin more than any other?

Learning from the Sessions – You – the Individual Nurse

As a junior psychologist, I was very interested in the experiences of staff working in the NHS. I read a lot about the impact of shift patterns and work type on individuals, and was fascinated to learn about the links between health behaviours and work type. For example poor working relationships can have an adverse impact on physical and mental health (Johansson et al., 2013). Although we believe that we are coping with the immediate stressor because we are able to manage in the moment, the research identified that the impact of the way we live our lives and the stressors we are exposed to may not be seen until much later in life (Johansson et al., 2013). Following a stressful episode, the body releases adrenaline, which affects the whole body, including the brain, but is fast-acting, leaving the brain after one minute. If the threat continues, cortisol is released, which, once in the brain, remains much longer, where it continues to affect brain cells. Over-secretion of stress hormones adversely affects brain function and sustained stress can damage the hippocampus, the part of the limbic brain, which is central to learning and memory (Wook Koo et al., 2010).

The capacity of the brain to deal with constant emotional challenge without any detrimental impact is limited (Weinstein and Ryan, 2011). The stream of 'input' whether it comes from a stressful shift, juggling the demands of work and home life or dealing with a challenging workplace can mean that we are more likely to be operating in a 'stressed mode'. Our bodies will be secreting more cortisol, which can have an adverse effect on mental and physical health (Frodl and O'Keane, 2013).

Modern-day stressors are interpreted by the body as a 'danger' during a perceived threat, for example struggling with a particularly difficult patient or relative, the adrenal glands immediately release adrenaline. As a stress hormone, it plays a major role in preparing the body for a fight-or-flight reaction (Brown, Varghese and McEwen, 2008). The cause of an increase in adrenaline secretion is often not an actual physical threat, but an imagined threat, such as the pressure to meet a work deadline. In order to cope with the cognitive demands of stress and the emotional arousal it can produce, we attempt to process whether the current event we are engaged in is a 'threat' (Figure 10.1) (Lazarus and Folkman, 1984). For a

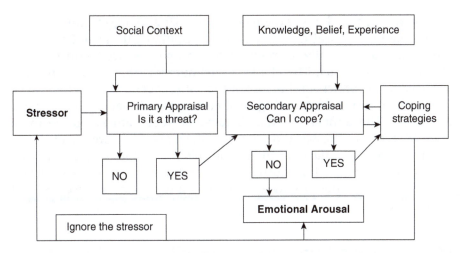

Figure 10.1 The stress and coping model.
Source: Lazarus and Folkman, 1984.

nurse, this might mean feeling overwhelmed by caring for a dependent patient and being aware that the patient's family needs emotional support. Nurses may process this as a potential 'threat' because they do not have the resources to cope.

In managing the situation or attempting to cope, disengaging emotionally is often a form of defence (Wallbank, 2007). In this way, the situation is less emotionally demanding but presents challenges to the delivery of care. Without giving of yourself and emotionally connecting, the compassionate care experience patients require is compromised. When the workplace becomes highly stressful for nurses, they are unable to keep 'giving of themself' without risking burnout, and there is an urgent need to protect their emotional self in order to avoid psychological difficulties (Wallbank, 2010). One community nurse described this as 'knocking on the door with a sponge', praying that the patient did not answer as she had nothing left to give.

Operating in a stressed mode results in slower functioning and reduced effectiveness. This is manifested in lateness, absence, relationship difficulties, impaired decision-making, lack of motivation, feeling overwhelmed, reluctance to engage, burnout and compassion fatigue (not having the capacity to care) (Wallbank and Robertson, 2010). The impact of staff experiencing such levels of stress contributes to an increase in the number of mistakes and 'near misses', and a reduction in the capacity of staff to think critically and make decisions (Firth-Cozens and Payne, 1999).

What can nurses do?

The research and my experience of working alongside nurses have shown me how critical it is to slow down thinking, to disrupt the stress mode that automatically takes over when people are faced with the situations outlined earlier. The challenge for nurses is that usually they are attracted to the profession because of their strong desire to care for others. They gain pleasure from giving of themselves and making things right for others. The difficulty is that because of your nature you are more vulnerable to the stresses and strains of the work. You care about others and the impact you have on them, and this means the work affects you. Managing and supporting yourself and your own reaction to the work you are involved in is often overlooked, yet is an integral part of the emotional work you do.

Managing and Supporting Yourself

So what does this look like in reality, and what can you do to support yourself? First, think about your own boundaries. From the number of times I have heard nurses tell me about how much above and beyond they give to their own workplace environments, I am convinced that the NHS only functions because of this goodwill. Indeed, the RCN employment survey (2013) reported that 66 per cent of the 9754 nurses who responded regularly work extra unpaid hours. The risk here is that this way of working can lead to burnout, especially if it becomes an accepted norm of your workplace rather than a choice you make. The compulsion to work later than your shift finish time, come in on your day off and give up your annual leave needs to be resisted. It is a strong driver for you as you want to help and support, but you also need to think about your overall capacity to work over a career, not just in the here and now. You need your days off to gain some perspective, to recharge and restore your sense of normality, which is highly protective. It also means you are able to give time to building relationships with friends and family which help protect you in your work. One of the most consistent protectors against stress is social support (Thoits, 2011).

One of the benefits of the restorative supervision sessions are that they prompt participants to think about their own needs and well-being. For example participants have started weight-loss programmes, pursued education programmes and/or made decisions about their work–life balance. Working in a demanding role where you care for others often leaves little time to focus on yourself. The sessions raise awareness that by taking care of yourself you can be a better carer for others. If carers are unwell or feeling overwhelmed by their own situation, then they are unlikely to provide the best care.

Learning from the Sessions – Thinking about the Patient Experience

The popularity of the Internet as a diagnostic tool for patients and their families and the rise in expectations that comes from an era of less respect for professionals (Lateef, 2011) have resulted in a change in the nature of the nurse–patient relationship. On one hand, patients are often at their most vulnerable and want to be cared for, and on the other they are less likely to heed advice and accept instructions.

An understanding of behavioural psychology and how to de-escalate situations is invaluable. I often heard from individuals in sessions how a low-key event with a patient or family turned into a full-blown issue because the family or patient misunderstood what was said. When we are in an anxious state as a patient or a patient's family member, our capacity to hear, reflect and respond appropriately is reduced. We hear the words, but somehow they are filtered through our own concerns, which translate them into something completely different. Patients are more likely to interpret behaviour or body language negatively when they have high levels of anxiety (Butow et al., 2002). If this is combined with a tired and overworked nurse, it is a recipe for misunderstanding and disappointment for all concerned.

Finding opportunities through supervision to express how you are managing your workload, how you have found particular care experiences or the difficulties you are experiencing can be useful in supporting you to become more resilient to these experiences in the future. The next section gives some examples from practice in the form of case studies to help you gain a better understanding of how the restorative sessions work.

Learning Points

➤ We can all support our colleagues in a restorative way, though we need to move from problem-solving to active listening.

➤ Helping people to think about how they can solve their own problems can be very powerful.

➤ If you need to offer support to a colleague, remember that sometimes silence is as powerful as the words of advice you want to share.

➤ A supportive network of colleagues and family is highly protective against stress (Firth-Cozens and Payne, 1999). Offering to spend time with colleagues sharing experiences away from the complexities of a shift may be supportive for you and your colleagues.

Case Study 1: **Sarah – Learning to Deal with Someone in a Restorative Way**

Walking into the ward, I could see a nurse whom I met regularly for restorative supervision sessions, looking concerned. She ushered me into the sluice urgently as if she had something secret to tell me. We had walked over 20 metres through the ward, and she had yet to let go of my arm. Once in the privacy of the sluice, she broke down. It had been an awful morning for her, having to nurse several terminally ill patients. Things were difficult at home; I knew this from our previous sessions, but we were not scheduled to meet for another few weeks.

Once she had told me, her calmness returned, but she looked shattered. I told her that it sounded like she was having an awful morning and that she was doing well to hold it together. There had been some difficulties with a member of staff having to go home sick, so the ward was short-staffed as well. I asked her why she had not telephoned and requested cover, and she responded that she thought she could cope. I listened as she explained, and as she was sharing her experiences, she began asking herself, 'Why did I think it was going to be an easy shift? Why didn't I ring for help earlier in the day?' Over a number of sessions with Sarah, she was able to reflect on her way of surviving shifts. She was able to consider why she felt that expressing her needs left her feeling vulnerable and not 'good enough' rather than seeing the reality, where she was at risk of burnout.

The role of the supervisor was to listen to Sarah explain how she was undertaking her job, and provide a safe space for the discussion to become productive and focus on what might be different. The supervisor also encourages a change in thinking about how to work. Given that the sessions were likely to challenge Sarah's current approach it was important that she felt safe with the supervisor so she could hear these challenges as constructive and not as criticism. Undertaking training to become an effective supervisor is important to the success of the sessions.

Although the early pilot work was not designed to improve working relationships, this has been one of its unintended positive consequences. The impact of working with other professionals, whether as part of the team or external to the team or workplace, has been significant. Through the sessions, as supervisees are able to process their own experiences more constructively, they appear to have less need to focus on themselves and their own difficulties. This seems to leave them more open to the needs of other people in their team, and they want to be helpful, more supportive or more challenging in an appropriate way of others in the team (Wallbank and Woods, 2012). This positive behaviour was also observed by colleagues and managers who had not been involved in the supervision programme. It is important to bear in mind that the individuals were

Case Study 2: **Simon – Impact of Restorative Supervision on Teams**

I was working with a group of doctors and nurses who worked in the field of child protection. They reported that a lack of teamwork and unclear roles were causing significant issues for each member of the team. Child protection work is complex, emotionally challenging and generates high levels of anxiety because the decisions the team make have serious implications for the families involved. The team was professionally led by others outside of the team, and there was no team manager as this was not felt to be a necessary role.

A number of unhelpful behaviours were occurring in the team, with individuals submitting late reports; typing their own versions of reports so as not to be associated with the reports written by others; aggressive behaviour (shouting, slamming doors and so on) and passive aggressive behaviour (not turning up to meetings, not talking in meetings, taking issues outside of the team without talking to the team). Although supervising members of the team individually resolved a number of the issues, bringing the team together as whole to understand each other's needs was the only way to deal with the more complex issues.

It soon became apparent during the meeting that a lack of a local leader meant that no one individual team member was being held to account for the work of the team. There were numerous misunderstandings of roles, deadlines and activity, and the team was not working well. Although it was clear the team would be better off with a leader, the capacity of the team to think about this and make a clear decision had been impaired by the difficulty of the work. All the team members described how the lack of a leader was making their individual roles difficult, but they were seemingly unable to think beyond the immediate problem.

Through the restorative supervision sessions, the team members were able to build better working relationships with each other and express what they needed to enable them to think about their work more clearly. Developing an understanding of each other's roles and eventually appointing a leader enabled the team to move on together and agree a set of clear objectives.

not behaving in a deliberately 'difficult' way prior to the sessions; it was more that they were overwhelmed by their own experiences and unable to think beyond that.

Positive relationships inside and outside your team can improve your capacity to think and care for the patients you are responsible for. Extensive research has been conducted on teamwork and the protective or detrimental effect it can have on patient safety (Maynard, Marshall and Dean, 2012) and patient outcomes (Auerbach et al., 2012). This is important in the processes the team undertakes and the relationships within that team.

Internal Relationships

An important element of good teamwork which emerged in the sessions is clarity of purpose. Job role conflict and ambiguity ('I thought
that was my responsibility' and 'I am unclear about what my role is in
this team') were the most frequently reported difficulties in the sessions.
This was often because of the configuration of the team and/or individuals working on tasks which had not been allocated fairly, the absence of
leaders, and confusion among the team arising from individuals coming
together across a care pathway, but managed and professionally led by
others.

Role ambiguity has been shown to reduce personal accomplishments,
whereas agreeableness and emotional stability increase personal accomplishments (Ghorpade, Lackritz and Singh, 2011). Agreeableness (a personality trait which indicates desire to please) is directly correlated with
career progression and reduced family–work conflict (Wille, De Fruyt and
Feys, 2012). During the sessions, it was apparent that even those individuals who usually displayed a high level of agreeableness were less likely to
want to 'please' or agree with others, perhaps due to their working environment. The desire to volunteer or to go above and beyond was significantly diminished where stress and burnout scores were high, and this had
an impact on the workplace. The fewer people who volunteered, the more
managers would put pressure on those who did to undertake additional
tasks.

Feeling connected to the organisation you work in by understanding how the aims and objectives affect the care you provide is protective
against the stresses and strains of the job. Knowing that what you do does
not just matter to you, the patients and their families, but to the entire
organisation, gives you the sense of purpose needed to carry you through
even the toughest of days. Not having that purpose in an organisation can
mean workforce dissatisfaction is high, as the following example shows:

> I can remember many years ago speaking with a director of nursing regarding
> the ideas I had about supporting staff in their workplace. This senior nurse said,
> 'The thing we have to decide, Sonya, is are we here for the patients or for the
> staff?' At the time, as a junior researcher I could not find the words to respond,
> probably because I did not understand this mindset. Surely, if an organisa-
> tion was not able to provide a supportive context for its staff, then those staff
> would be unable to provide that support their patients? As I reflect now, I can
> see the nursing director was overwhelmed; there I stood reminding him of
> the importance of looking after the staff, when looking after the patients was
> a difficult enough task in itself. Compartmentalising the system in terms of

those who needed the care and those who provided it was his way of protecting himself. If the nurses providing the care also needed to be thought about, when would there be time for that to happen? It was simpler, and 'safer' for him, in a psychological sense, not to think about it. During the research and supervision sessions, I have often encountered this approach to self-protection among practitioners. Now, though, I know how to support staff to recognise their vulnerability.

Conclusion

Restorative supervision sessions are one research-based solution to managing the pressures of work which can be incorporated into your working life to help maintain your resilience. The programme aims to raise awareness about the inherent risks in practice and how to find ways to work on being more resilient. You can use a number of strategies without the need for formalised sessions.

> Build your life outside of work – ensure that work does not dominate you every day as this has been shown to be most protective against stress.

> Protect your work–life balance – remember to top yourself up with positive energy gained from good experiences outside of work daily.

> Build strong networks within your workplace and with individuals doing similar work in other organisations – it is highly protective against stress and excellent for learning.

> Find others who can share and discuss your work experiences with you so that you are able to process them while being supported emotionally – think of peer supervision or action learning sets as a support for you.

> Find a balance to the emotional demands at work by involving yourself with tasks that you enjoy – compassion satisfaction (the pleasure you derive from work) is highly protective.

> Notice when you are becoming less energetic or that things are getting on top of you. Approach your line manager or your colleagues for support and be clear about what you need from others.

Nursing is an occupation which makes emotional as well as physical demands on you as an individual. To improve your capacity to cope with these over time, you need to be able to process your experiences so that they do not accumulate and cause you to be less emotionally connected. Although you may be able to cope in the moment, a stressful life over a sustained period has negative physical and psychological effects, which in turn will reduce compassion. Engaging in restorative supervision enables individuals and groups to create a place where experiences can be processed, functioning and behaviour can be challenged productively and solutions reached in order to improve long-term capacity to think (Wallbank, 2010). Improving your capacity to think and make decisions even in the face of difficult and complex patient care will enable you to continue to deliver compassionate care as you remain firmly engaged with patients and their needs.

References

Auerbach, A., N. Sehgal, M. Belgen et al. (2012) 'Effects of a Multicentre Teamwork and Communication Programme on Patient Outcomes: Results from the Triad for Optimal Patient Safety (TOPS) Project', *British Medical Journal Quality and Safety,* 21(2): 118–26.

Brown, E., F. Varghese and B. McEwen (2004) 'Association of Depression with Medical Illness: Does Cortisol Play a Role?', *Biological Psychiatry,* 55(1): 1–9.

Butow, P., R. Brown and S. Coger et al. (2002) 'Oncologists' Reactions to Cancer Patients' Verbal Cues', *Psycho-Oncology,* 11(1): 47–58.

Chartered Institute of Personnel Development (CIPD) Department of Health (1993) *A Vision for the Future: The Nursing, Midwifery and Health Visiting Contribution to Healthcare* (London: The NHS Management Executive).

Department of Health (2013) 'Using Restorative Supervision to Improve Practice and Safeguarding Decisions', www.gov.uk/government/uploads/system/uploads/attachment_data/file/209911/S15_Restorative_Supervision_Surrey_EISCS_V121211.pdf.

Firth-Cozens, J. and R. Payne (1999) *Stress in Health Professionals Psychological and Organisations Causes and Interventions* (Chichester, NY: John Wiley & Sons).

Frodl, T. and V. O'Keane (2013) 'How Does the Brain Deal with Cumulative Stress? A Review with Focus on Developmental Stress, HPA Axis Function and Hippocampal Structure in Humans', *Neurobiology of Disease,* 52: 24–37.

Ghorpade J, J. Lackritz and G. Singh (2011) 'Personality as a Moderator of the Relationship Between Role Conflict, Role Ambiguity, and Burnout', *Journal of Applied Social Psychology,* 41(6): 1275–98.

Johansson, L., X. Guo, T. Hällström et al. (2013) 'Common Psychosocial Stressors in Middle-aged Women Related to Longstanding Distress and Increased Risk of Alzheimer's Disease: A 38-year Longitudinal Population Study', *British Medical Journal Open,* 30 September, http://bmjopen.bmj.com/content/3/9/e003142.abstract.

Kadushin, A. (1992) *Clinical Supervisor* (New York: Haworth).

Kahneman, D. (2012) *Thinking, Fast and Slow* (New York: Penguin Books) Part 1: The Lazy Controller, p. 39.

Lateef, F. (2011) 'Patient Expectations and the Paradigm Shift of Care in Emergency Medicine', *Journal of Emergency Trauma Shock,* 4(2): 163–7.

Lazarus, R. S. and S. Folkman (1984) *Stress, Appraisal and Coping* (New York: Springer).

Maynard, T., D. Marshall and M. Dean (2012) 'Crew Resource Management and Teamwork Training in Healthcare: A Review of the Literature and Recommendations for how to Leverage such Interventions to Enhance Patient Safety', in Leonard H. Friedman, Grant T. Savage, Jim Goes (eds) *Annual Review of Health Care Management: Strategy and Policy Perspectives on Reforming Health Systems (Advances in Health Care Management*, Vol. 13) (Emerald Group Publishing Limited) 59–91.

Proctor, B. (1986) 'Supervision – A Co-operative Exercise in Accountability', in M. Marken and M. Payne (eds) *Enabling and Ensuring: Supervision in Practice, National Bureau and Council for Education and Training in Youth and Community Work* (Leicester: National Youth Bureau) 21–3.

Royal College of Nursing (RCN) (2013) Employment Survey 2013, Royal College of Nursing, London, www2.rcn.org.uk/__data/assets/pdf_file/0005/541292/ Employment_Survey_2013_004_503_FINAL_100214.pdf.

Schaufeli, W. and A. B. Bakker (2004) 'Job Demands, Job Resources, and Their Relationship with Burnout and Engagement: A Multi-sample Study', *Journal of Organizational Behaviour*, 25(3): 293–315.

Stamm, B. (2010) *The Concise PROQOL Manual*, 2nd edn (Pocatello, ID: ProQOL. org), http://proqol.org/uploads/ProQOL_Concise_2ndEd_12-2010.pdf.

Tarrant, T. and C. Sabo (2011) 'Role Conflict, Role Ambiguity and Job Satisfaction in Nurse Executives', *Nursing Administration Quarterly*, 34(1): 72–82.

Thoits, P. (2011) 'Mechanisms Linking Social Ties and Support to Physical and Mental Health', *Journal of Health & Social Behavior*, 52(2): 145–61.

Wallbank, S. (2007) Impact of Miscarriage, Stillbirth and Loss on Doctors, Nurses and Midwives, PhD thesis, Leicester University.

Wallbank, S. (2010) 'Effectiveness of Individual Clinical Supervision for Midwives and Doctors in Stress Reduction: Findings from a Pilot Study', *Evidence-based Midwifery*, 8(2): 28–34.

Wallbank, S. (2012) 'Health Visitors' Needs – National Perspectives from the Restorative Clinical Supervision Programme', *Community Practitioner*, 85(11), 26–9.

Wallbank, S. (2013a) 'Recognizing Stressors and Using Restorative Supervision to Support a Healthier Maternity Workforce', *Evidence Based Midwifery*, www.rcm.org.uk/learning-and-career/learning-and-research/ebm-articles/ recognising-stressors-and-using-restorative.

Wallbank, S. (2013b) 'Reflecting on Leadership in Health Visiting and the Restorative Model of Supervision', *Journal of Health Visiting*, 1(3): 2–4.

Wallbank, S. and N. Robertson (2010) 'Midwife and Nurse Responses to Miscarriage, Stillbirth and Neonatal Death', *Evidence-based Midwifery*, 6: 100–6.

Wallbank, S. and N. Robertson (2013) 'Predictors of Staff Stress in Response to Professionally Experienced Miscarriage, Stillbirth and Neonatal Loss', *International Journal of Nursing*, 50(8): 1090–7.

Wallbank, S. and G. Woods (2012) 'A Healthier Health Visiting Workforce: Findings from the Restorative Supervision Programme', *Community Practitioner*, 85(11): 20–3.

Weinstein, N. and R. Ryan (2011) 'A Self-Determination Theory Approach to Understanding Stress Incursion and Responses', *Stress and Health*, 27: 4–17.

Wille, B., F. De Fruyt and M. Feys (2012) 'Big Five Traits and Intrinsic Success in the New Career Era: A 15-Year Longitudinal Study on Employability and Work–Family Conflict', *Applied Psychology*, 62: 124–56.

Wook Koo, J., S. Russo, D. Ferguson et al. (2010) 'Nuclear Factor-κB Is a Critical Mediator of Stress-impaired Neurogenesis and Depressive Behavior', *Biological Sciences – Neuroscience*, 107(6): 2669–74.

11

Compassion, Emotional Labour and Public Service in the United States

Sharon Mastracci

Introduction: The Link between Compassion and Emotional Labour

Evidence on emotional labour from studies of emergency responders in the United States can inform research on compassion in UK public service organisations. Emotional labour scholarship informs the study of compassion because, contrary to the notion that 'compassion costs nothing' (Sawbridge, this volume, quoting CQC, 2011), emotional labour – the effort to suppress or elicit emotions in oneself and/or patients and clientele – is the cost of compassion. In order to exhibit compassionate care, caregivers must engage in mental processes to tune out whatever stressors may be present, engage fully with the patient/client, and truly feel – or at least appear to feel – compassion for the other person. Emotional labour is the mental process by which this is done. In their examination of compassion in organisations, Atkins and Parker (2012) note that evidence on emotional labour 'in the helping professions suggests that encouraging people to become more compassionate without considering the associated self-regulatory demands can lead to staff burnout and turnover' (p. 524). This may be why Rynes et al. (2012) observe that 'care and compassion ... may emerge where they are least expected and may well be endangered where they are most expected' (2012: 503). Among healthcare workers where care and compassion would be expected, evidence suggests that care and compassion have become endangered (Bevan and Hood, 2006) as healthcare workers increasingly suffer burnout and the negative effects of staff turnover: 'Nowhere is this more apparent than in the English National Health Service (NHS) where recent damning reports have exposed appalling standards of personal care and neglect' (Mannion, 2014: 1). The Francis Report (2013) catalogued the 'appalling standards of personal care' at one NHS Trust and concluded that care and compassion had indeed become endangered: 'Healthcare needs to have a culture of caring, commitment, and compassion ... it cannot be assumed that such a culture is shared by all who provide healthcare services to patients' (2013: 1360). The Francis Report also speculates on why care and compassion became endangered: 'People come into the professions with compassion and interpersonal skills but ... when they're subjected to the pressures of a modern care environment they can become inured to suffering [which] is a human reaction to a high stress, high pressure job' (2013: 1376). If care workers in high-stress jobs are encouraged to become more compassion-ate, without considering the emotional labour demands needed to do so, then poor care, burnout and turnover can arise. Emotional labour suffuses care work: 'Human services [is] a high emotional-labour occupation with an associated high risk of burnout' (Lilius, 2012: 569), and an inability to account for the importance of emotional labour diminishes the effective-ness of any steps taken to increase compassion in organisations.

This chapter is organised as follows: in the next section, I review the roots of our understanding of emotional labour in public services. Despite its origins in the Progressive Era, public administration and public service scholarship reflects scientific management principles of the early twen-tieth century rather than the principles of humanism, which developed in the field of social work in the United States (Stivers, 2000). The next section also contains an overview of emotional labour research, including our work with public servants in the US. The third section is comprised of an analysis of transcripts from interviews with emergency responders to examine compassion in organisations, using the Gioia Methodology (Gioia, Corley and Hamilton, 2012). In the fourth section, I discuss the findings of the analysis of compassion in emergency response personnel, including a proposition resulting from this analysis that could be used in future research. Finally, the fifth section discusses conclusions and direc-tions for further research, including a discussion of several instances in the Francis Report (2013), where compassion is underscored as integral to providing high-quality healthcare.

Background on Emotional Labour Scholarship in Public Service

Early American scholarship on the role of individuals in organisations is rooted in scientific management principles, which arose from the Industrial Revolution and mass production processes, where individuals are characterised as part of a larger production process, as cogs in a greater machine. American management theorist Frederick Taylor, whose name is synonymous with scientific management, captures these principles in an archetypal statement: 'In the past, man has been first, in the future the system must be first' (1911: 2). In this view, the characteristics of individuals do not matter in the workplace. Workers are interchangeable, and only their objective output matters to the organisation. The role of the individual worker in scientific management is consistent with the role of the individual in Max Weber's 'ideal type' bureaucracy, which 'develops the more perfectly the more the bureaucracy is dehumanized, the more completely it succeeds in eliminating from official business love, hatred, and all purely personal, irrational, and emotional elements which escape calculation' (1948: 973). Taken together, the individual worker is subordinate to the system in capital-intensive mass production processes (Taylor) and also in the production of services delivered by the ideal bureaucracy (Weber). Public services, being services and not tangible goods, are not produced in a factory, but rather by people in organisations. Weber's ideal bureaucracy provided the blueprint for early American theorists of public service, who imported Weber into government at the same time as the demands for a professionalised public service grew during the Progressive Era. Not everyone at that time, however, applied efficiency ideals from the factory floor to the public servant's desktop. A critique of scientific management principles is found among scholars taking a Post-Fordist, humanistic approach to the individual in organisations, a holistic approach to theorising about the worker as a whole person, not a cog in a mass production process. One example of this critique comes from Jane Addams, who worked alongside municipal reformers during the turn of the last century and lamented that they 'fix their attention so exclusively on methods that they fail to consider the final aims of city government' (Stivers, 2009: 94). Municipal reformers – proto-public administration practitioners during the Progressive Era – were too occupied with counting output to capture what counted, in Jane Addams' view. Decades later, Dwight Waldo notes little had changed: 'The formal analysis of organizations without regard to the purposes that inspire them [is] but a tedious elabouration of the insignificant' (1948: 211). Working alongside management theorists deeply influenced by Weberian ideals, Mary Parker Follett observed, 'Orders come from the work not work from the orders ... it is a fallacy to think that an order gets its validity from consent. It gets its validity long before that, from the whole process to which both order-giver and order-receiver have contributed' (1949: 31). Voices from the scientific management school were influential in the development of the relatively new scholarly field studying public services and administration during this time, resulting in contemporary theory that still reflects its positivist origins; a theory that does not make room for emotions. Where the individual is examined at all, a worker is characterised as a set of measurable knowledge, skills, and abilities, or human capital endowments;

and women as employees were rarely mentioned at all. In production processes requiring physical labour, the individual worker possesses a set of physical attributes that determine how well she or he can do the job. Knowledge workers possess a set of cognitive abilities that determine her or his ability to do the job. What of public servants and care workers? Production processes that do not account for the whole worker – emotions and all – fail to capture characteristics crucial to the work of public servants, and entirely fail to fit the reality faced by care workers. As public administration scholar Robert Kramer observes, 'Governance is more than the machinery of public administration, and more than the machinery of impartial cost-benefit analysis ... Human relationships are at the heart of governance ... all public service is people ... Human relationships are the DNA of governance' (2003: 2).

Performance evaluations and job descriptions fail to capture the human dimensions of public service (Guy and Newman, 2004; Mastracci, Newman and Guy, 2006) and are therefore stuck in an image of work forged during the industrial age by management scientists blind to the human processes by which work gets done. The preoccupation with cognitive processes 'can lead to theory and research that portrays organization members as cognitive stick figures whose behavior is unaffected by emotions' (Mowday and Sutton, 1993: 197). Scholars of public administration and public service maintain just such an image of work: 'At its inception, public administration paid homage to the "god" of science ... The developing field of management science prescribed principles of management that emphasized efficiency over all else. In its purest sense, the god of efficiency ... is simple, clear-cut, and short-sighted' (Guy, 2003: 643, 647). Madden et al. (2012) concur: 'We have relied on models of organizations as machines for over a hundred years. It is time to articulate organizations as reflections of our best selves – as communities where compassion, support, and positive energy are expected, natural, and normal' (2012: 704). Camilla Stivers concludes that the aversion to examining factors like compassion in organisations as natural and normal is deliberate and gendered: 'Part of the reason for public administration's preference for scientific administration over the values that animated municipal housekeeping – for efficiency over caring – was the threat to municipal reformers posed by the gender accusations of party politicians: specifically, the risk to their masculinity that lay in associating themselves with women's benevolent activities' (2000: 125). Associating care and compassion with femininity – and something to be avoided – goes back at least as far as the third century BC, when 'the Stoics often portrayed compassion as a weakness and a feminine trait' (Rynes et al., 2012: 506). Carroll (2001: 103) demonstrates how 'the American system of public administration and government can clearly trace its beginnings to the English system of government'; whether the gendered bias against care and compassion is uniquely American, however, he does not say.

Emotional labour is the effort to suppress inappropriate emotions and/or elicit appropriate emotions within oneself or in another person, where 'appropriate' and 'inappropriate' are dictated by the demands of the job. Emotional labour is so integral to some jobs that to fail to engage in emotional labour is to fail to do the job. A social worker cannot laugh at her clients' circumstances. A police officer cannot show fear to criminal suspects. An emergency responder (paramedic) cannot panic or recoil from a patient's gruesome injuries as she arrives on the scene of an accident. Emotional labour research largely began with Arlie Russell Hochschild's study of flight attendants, where their performance of emotional labour fostered repeat business and benefitted their employer's bottom line. Hochschild underscores the transactional nature of this effort: 'Emotional labour is sold for a wage and therefore has exchange value ... it is bought on one hand and sold on the other' (1983: 7). Hochschild introduced emotional labour to the study of organisations by sociologists and management theorists. Among scholars of public services and administration, Guy and Newman's 2004 paper is the first to examine emotional labour. They hypothesise that the gender wage gap is attributable to unpaid emotional labour and examine pay, job descriptions and job attributes of state employees in Illinois, New Jersey, Oregon and Florida in three selected listings in the Career Service Class: driver license examiner, food inspector and social service counsellor. They find that although the food inspector earns almost as much as the social service counsellor, few qualifications are required for the food inspector position; almost no demands for interpersonal skills are required; and more than three-fourths – 83 per cent – of jobholders are men. In contrast, both the driver license examiner and the social service counsellor require significantly more interpersonal interaction and emotional labour, and almost two-thirds of all driver license examiners are women and more than three-fourths of all social service counsellors are women. To the extent that occupational segregation by gender among public employees in England reflects what Guy and Newman find among public servants in the United States, then their findings inform the study of emotional labour in the UK as well. Guy and Newman conclude that unpaid and taken-for-granted emotional labour exerted by female public employees accounts for the overrepresentation of women in certain jobs – occupational segregation by gender – which in turn accounts for the gender wage gap found in these and other occupations. They call for further research on the emotional components of occupations: 'As we move further and further away from organizations

that are designed to operate assembly lines, we must devise new structures that capture today's work and skill requirements ... Making emotional labour visible is the first step, making it compensable is the next'
(Guy and Newman, 2004: 296).

In *Emotional Labour: Putting the Service in Public Service* (Guy, Newman
and Mastracci, 2008), we took that next step, expanding upon Guy and
Newman (2004) to further develop the concept of emotional labour in
public service jobs. We addressed several questions: What is emotional
labour? Who engages in it? Is it specific to a department? A job? To certain people? The latter questions are important to answer, given the
habit of equating emotional labour with care work and equating both
with female workers. Women are disproportionately employed in caring
professions, and by essentialising care to gender, employers and society
take for granted that women will engage in even extensive emotional
labour without acknowledging it, much less compensating for it (Grant
and Patil, 2012). We surveyed and interviewed workers at three different
agencies and departments in state and local government: a state-level
department of corrections, a county office of Public Guardian (children
and family services), and municipal-level workers in a 911 dispatch
centre – akin to 999 call centres in England. We compiled data from
more than 300 surveys (roughly 100 per site with response rates between
42 and 51 per cent) and dozens of interviews. Our three sites differed
in theoretically important ways – in ways that would affect the nature
of emotional labour demanded on the job (Lilius, 2012). For instance,
while corrections and family services workers engage with citizens and
clients face-to-face, 911 dispatchers interact strictly voice-to-voice. The
duration of interactions varies by site as well – while the 'relationships'
between callers and 911 dispatchers last mere minutes, corrections workers and Public Guardian staff can know their clients for days, months,
even years. Likewise, although corrections workers and Public Guardian
staff often know what happened to different prisoners or wards of the
state, 911 dispatchers usually never know the outcomes of their calls
unless they make follow-up inquiries with individual emergency responders. The nature of these relationships varies by site, too – although 911
dispatchers and Public Guardian staff try to build trust relationships
with their clients, corrections workers operate entirely in an environment of distrust. Likewise, whereas the former are perceived as victims
in crisis who need help, the latter are convicted criminals who need to
be controlled in the best interests of public safety. Through analysis of
interview transcripts and survey data, we arrive at several conclusions.
First, emotional labour is fundamental to quality public service and is the
product of both face-to-face and voice-to-voice interaction. Emotional
labour involves both eliciting an emotional state in another person

and/or managing one's own desired and undesired emotions, all for the purpose of doing one's job. Second, both male and female employees engage in emotional labour. Women do not exert more emotional labour than do their male colleagues, although the nature of emotional labour differs between women and men; in other words, emotional labour demands are dictated by the job, not the sex of the worker. Third, both new employees and long-tenured ones engage in emotional labour; neither exerts more or less emotional labour. Emotional labour is not specific to an agency or department; it is located in the job and not the jobholder; the nature of emotional labour will vary by job, however, and some jobs involve more emotional labour than others. Fourth, emotions in the workplace are not antithetical to professionalism. On-the-job emotion regulation – emotional labour – takes skill, significant effort and is key to getting the job done. An additional contribution of our first book was to characterise high emotional labour jobs as not only exhausting but also potentially fulfilling. We further concluded that organisations should acknowledge emotional labour in job descriptions, hiring procedures, training and professional development materials, employee assistance and wellness programs, performance evaluations, and compensation practices. In Chapter 8, it has already been described as a role requirement for nurses.

Once we put emotional labour on the radar, we then asked: *How* do public servants engage in it? In *Emotional Labour: Working on the Razor's Edge* (Mastracci, Newman and Guy, 2012), we conducted in-depth interviews with experienced emergency responders in three urban areas: Chicago, Denver and Miami. Our deliberate choice of high-intensity occupations like those in emergency response was inspired by Carol Gilligan's path-breaking book *In a Different Voice* (1982), in which she studied the gendered nature of moral decision-making by interviewing women considering abortions. The decision was obviously not 'random' or 'representative' of all decisions that a woman will face, but was one that allowed her to capture the strategies and approaches that women take when making moral judgements. Gilligan reasoned that if there were any decisions that would betray a woman's moral calculus – this was one. Likewise, we reasoned that if there was any type of public service that would reveal workers' strategies and approaches to exercising emotional labour, crisis response would be it. We asked: In an instant and faced with panicked and traumatised victims, how do workers size up a situation and decide how to proceed? How do they establish trust and elicit cooperation? How do they use discretion in different situations? Answers to these questions matter – not only to provide more tangible guidance to public managers after alerting the field to the phenomenon of emotional labour, but also because of the cognitive cost of emotional labour. When one is deliberately suppressing an unwanted emotion or eliciting a desired emotion – in other words, engaging in emotional labour – fewer resources are available for cognitive processing. Mistakes can be made on the job when engaging in emotional labour. Therefore, we argued, it is crucial to understand the emotional labour demands on workers. Experimental psychologists Richards and Gross (1999) directed study subjects *not to react* to disturbing images of auto accidents that they were shown. These subjects consistently performed poorly on tests of working memory compared to subjects who were not directed to suppress their reactions. Functional magnetic resonance imaging (fMRI) of study subjects' brains illustrated that the activation of certain areas during emotion suppression left fewer resources available to apply to cognitive tasks like working memory tests (Gross and Thompson, 2007; Pugh, Groth and Hennig-Thurau, 2011; Richards and Gross; 1999; Sheppes and Gross, 2011). This is not to say that emotions obscure reasoning; in fact, 'there has been a growing understanding by neuroscientists that emotions are not separate from reason and that, contrary to earlier beliefs, emotions often enhance reasoning abilities' (Rynes et al., 2012: 507). Suppression of emotion, however, draws resources away from cognitive task completion.

We conclude that to adequately hire, train, develop and evaluate workers on the basis of performance, we must address the whole job, not just its cognitive aspects. Workers must be trained and supported in their jobs if they are required to suppress, control and elicit their own and others' emotions as the job demands. Employers must prepare employees for emotional labour demands and equip them with the skills and resources necessary to manage their own and others' emotions as their work situations demand – and reward them for doing it well. Self-care strategies such as reflective practice and post-incident critical incident stress debriefings (CISDs) help first responders address the emotional labour demands of their jobs. We found several answers to our 'how' question. First, emergency responders effectively engage in extreme levels of emotional labour through execution of well-planned standard operating procedures, standing orders, and intense, repeated training designed to make decision-making almost automatic. Second, uniforms take away the individual characteristics of workers and turn them into generic responders, thereby emphasising authority while masking demographic differences. Workers become their role. Third, employers acknowledging the emotional dimensions of work and the emotional labour demands on their workers provide the context within which workers can engage in emotional labour and minimise risk of burnout. Finally, articulating 'how' highlights the actions and behaviours employers can target in job descriptions and performance evaluations to make emotional labour compensable.

Emergency Responders and Compassion

In this chapter, I investigate the presence or absence of compassion in emergency response by revisiting the interview transcripts from our 2012 book. We chose emergency response based on the high likelihood of its practitioners to exert emotional labour in intense, on-the-job situations. Respondents included police officers, firefighters, emergency medical technicians, crisis hotline workers, sexual assault nurse examiners, trauma nurses, medical examiners, public hospital administrators, and domestic violence and victim assistance workers. These employment situations are similar to the high-intensity conditions faced by nurses in NHS Trusts, and therefore what we learn from emergency responders can inform future research on compassion in the NHS.

Forty-three emergency responders were interviewed, resulting in nearly 50 hours of interview time logged by the researchers. Over their careers, our respondents had been called to hundreds of emergencies, including several notable crises: the 11 September 2001 attack on the World Trade Center in New York City, Hurricane Andrew in south Florida in 1992, Hurricane Katrina in New Orleans in 2005, the Columbine school shootings in 1999 and the 2010 earthquakes in Haiti. Interviews were recorded and transcribed, resulting in the 'word data' (Yanow and Schwartz-Shea, 2006: xix) upon which our results are based. Transcript analysis was also facilitated by use of the qualitative data analysis software package ATLAS.ti. Using respondent voices as expert testimony, we examine patterns of behaviour and decision-making in crisis response from the ground up, rather than imposing frameworks onto their narratives from the top down. As such, we make no claims with respect to random sampling of study participants or universal representation of their narratives because, in this study, 'concepts are embedded within a literature ... the attempt to specify them once and for all as universal constructs violates interpretive presuppositions about the historical locatedness of scholars and actors' (Yanow and Schwartz-Shea, 2006: xvii). (Our interview protocol is found in the appendix, p200.)

To examine compassion in emergency response, I employ semiotic clustering, also known as the Gioia Methodology (Gioia, Corley and Hamilton, 2012). This methodology allows me to take 'a systematic approach to new concept development and grounded theory articulation' (p. 15) and involves three steps: first, group respondent direct quotes into first-order concepts; second, organise concepts into second-order themes; and third, refine themes into broad dimensions. The 'systematic presentation of both a "first order" analysis (i.e.: an analysis using informant-centric terms and codes) and a "second order" analysis (i.e.: one using researcher-centric concepts, themes, and dimensions)' introduces methodological rigour into qualitative analysis (Gioia, Corley and Hamilton, 2012: 18). Theory firmly grounded in word data emanates from explaining relationships among the dimensions developed in step 3.

Findings from Qualitative Analysis

Figure 11.1 shows the results of three levels of analysis in the Gioia Methodology: First-order analysis 'tries to adhere faithfully to inform-ant terms'. Accordingly, the items in the first column in Figure 11.1 are direct quotes from respondents grouped by concept. Grouping respond-ent quotes is the first step, resulting in first-order concepts. In the sec-ond level of analysis, 'we start seeking similarities and differences among the many categories' (Gioia, Corley and Hamilton, 2012: 20). In step 2, I label the groupings from step 1. In step 3, 'we investigate whether it is possible to distill the emergent second-order themes even further' (2012: 20) and group second-order themes into aggregate dimensions. Explaining how aggregate dimensions interact results in theory grounded in word data.

Figure 11.1 is the three-column data structure prescribed by the Gioia Methodology, which illustrates the analytical steps taken to organise respondent quotes into themes and then into theoretical dimensions. The ultimate objective of the method is to explain the relationships among the aggregate dimensions, resulting in 'a vibrant inductive model that is grounded in the data (as exemplified by the data struc-ture), one that captures the informants' experience in theoretical terms' (Gioia, Corley and Hamilton, 2012: 22). Based on our prior research on emotional labour, I posit the following relationships among the three aggregate dimensions shown in Figure 11.1: in the context of highly visible and scrutinised work, given the public nature of the work and a sense of public ownership due to citizens' role as taxpayers, indi-vidual emergency responders employ organisational or individual self-preservation techniques in order to engage in emotional labour. Emotional labour is a combination of self-awareness and empathy. Self-awareness can be enhanced formally by employers that foster an envi-ronment to support the emotional labour demands on their employees, or informally by individuals emphasising task interdependency in their organisations (Grant and Patil, 2012; Madden et al., 2012). Employers can foster such an environment by recruiting and hiring individuals who are aware of their emotional responses at work and who can gauge their emotional status at any given time, and by implementing practices to cultivate emotional self-awareness and ongoing emotional manage-ment such as critical incident stress debriefings and self-care plans.

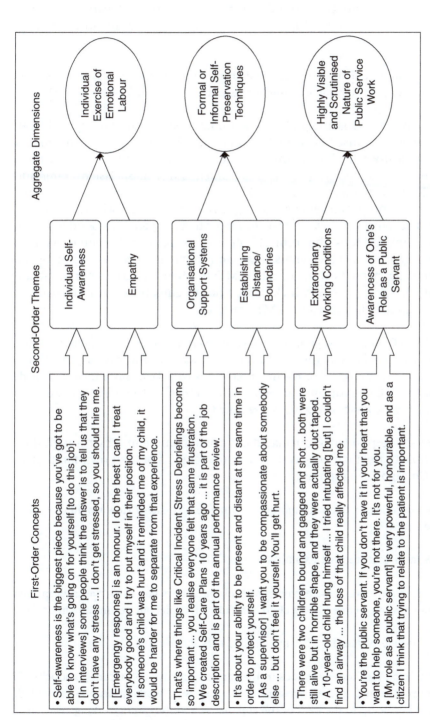

Figure 11.1 Data structure from direct quotes to themes to aggregate dimensions.

Organisations can purposefully cultivate an 'ethic of care' (Lawrence and Maitlis, 2012: 641). This theorised relationship results in the following proposition:

> Proposition 1: Public servants that demonstrate self-awareness and empathy will engage in emotional labour and express compassion for their clientele.

Self-awareness is integral to emotional labour and the expression of compassion because 'individuals will know "who they are" have a stronger sense of self-worth, hence, they will be less threatened and overwhelmed by another's suffering' (Atkins and Parker, 2012: 536). Hsieh, Yang and Fu (2011) also established a link between compassion and emotional labour: As compassion increased, cognitive dissonance – which is strongly related to burnout – was lower. Among our emergency responders, compassion mainly took the form of empathy for patients by public servants demonstrating self-awareness. Emotional labour enables compassion. An emergency medical technician (EMT) in Miami describes her first-hand experience as a patient, which caused her to empathise with her patients and ultimately informed her EMT practice:

> I had a C-section last year, and it was an emergency C-section, and nobody was telling me what was going on. I thought I was going to have a panic attack. I just started crying. For the first time, I was panicked. [Since then] I've made sure even if [the patient] is in cardiac arrest, I try to talk to them, because if you don't know what's going on, you're scared.

Several respondents articulated compassion and empathy through their principle to treat patients as if they were members of their own families, as this Chicago firefighter asks:

> How would you like your mother or father to be treated? How would *you* like to be treated?

His Miami counterpart explains:

> There's something about having a child that allows you to put yourself in their shoes; where before I had a child, it would affect me, but not in the same way.

And a police officer in Chicago echoes this sentiment:

> A woman had too many kids in the car and they weren't wearing seatbelts. Of course she gets into an accident. Well, they were working on one of the kids and I came up to the back of the ambulance and they were working away and I

caught a glimpse of the kid. At that time my kids were about that age and it hit me. I had to go back to the car and sit for a little bit. I was thinking, 'What if that was my kid?'

Compassion as empathy is found throughout the recommendations for the NHS in the Francis Report, for instance: 'Staff were encouraged to think about what they would want for themselves and their families as the standard for providing care' (2013: 1515). The Francis Report also cautions the NHS from taking compassion for granted, characterises compassion as a skill to be learned and encourages employers to recognise and compensate for the effort involved in providing compassionate care (2013: 1497):

> The aptitude and commitment of candidates for entry into nursing to provide basic hands-on care to patients should be tested by a minimum period of work experience, by aptitude testing and by nationally consistent practical training ... The specialist skills, commitment, and compassion needed for the nursing care of the elderly should be accorded the recognition they deserve by creation of a specialist registered status.

Conclusions: Compassion in Organisations

Compassion is not without cost. The cost of compassion is emotional labour: The effort to suppress or elicit emotions in oneself and/or patients and clientele. Emotional suppression draws resources away from cognitive tasks, meaning mistakes can be made. Encouraging healthcare workers to become more compassionate without considering the cost of emotional labour can lead to burnout and turnover (Atkins and Parker, 2012). Evidence from our research on emotional labour informs the scholarship on compassion in organisations by clarifying the concept of emotional labour and identifying how public servants engage in emotional labour in order to capture aspects of work that can provide organisational support for emotional labourers. Russell Mannion concludes 'organizational and cultural context can make an important difference in how care is delivered and experienced ... compassionate care does not occur in a vacuum and organizational context is particularly pertinent in shaping and mediating how care is delivered, experienced, and received' (2014: 2). Organisations can recruit for self-awareness and take steps to enhance employee self-awareness and empathy by emphasising the interrelatedness of tasks (Grant and Patil, 2012). Self-care programmes and critical incident stress debriefings, and reflective practice in general, all help care workers develop healthy boundaries so that they may engage in emotional labour without their work becoming all-consuming.

Appendix: Interview Protocol

1. When someone asks you to describe your job, what do you usually say?

2. In your line of work, do you feel a certain responsibility toward a particular group? If so, toward who or what?

3. Have you ever had an incident where your abilities or credibility was questioned? For instance, has anyone ever said to you:

   a. Do you have any idea what I'm going through?

   b. Aren't you a little young/old to be doing this?

   c. Do you have any idea what you're doing?

   d. You don't look/sound like a (firefighter, nurse, police officer, etc.)

      i. What happened?

      ii What did you do?

4. Have you ever had an incident when you had to bend or break the rules (think entirely outside the box, something came out of left field, etc.)? – when you had to suddenly change course, readjust or depart from standard operating procedure?

   a. What happened?

   b. What did you do?

5. Have you ever suffered your own crisis of confidence?

   a. What happened?

   b. What did you do?

6. Have you ever had a completely chaotic incident when it was up to you (there was no one else to turn to) to re-establish control? Alternatively, have you ever been called in to help someone else handle an incident?

   a. What happened?

   b. What did you do?

7. Is there a particular incident that sticks out in your mind when everything went wrong (hit the fan)?

   a. What happened?

   b. What did you do?

    c. What was the fallout?

    d. What role, if any, does this case play in the way you do your job now?

8. Is there a particular incident that sticks out in your mind, when everything went right?

    a. What happened?

    b. What did you do?

    c. What was the fallout?

    d. What role, if any, does this case play in the way you do your job now?

References

Atkins, P.W.B. and Sharon K. Parker (2012) 'Understanding Individual Compassion in Organizations: The Role of Appraisals and Psychological Flexibility', *Academy of Management Review*, 37(4): 524–46.

Bevan, G. and C. Hood (2006) 'What's Measured Is What Matters: Targets and Gaming in the English Public Healthcare System', *Public Administration*, 84(3): 517–38.

Care Quality Commission (CQC) (UK) (2011) 'Dignity and Nutrition Inspection Programme: National Overview', www.cpa.org.uk, accessed 2 June 2014.

Carroll, J. (2001) 'Roots to Branches: Tracing the Foundations of American Public Administration in Medieval England', in Ali Farazmand (ed.) *Handbook of Comparative and Public Administration*, 2nd edn (New York: Marcel Dekker) Chapter 8.

Follett, M. P. (1949) *Freedom and Coordination: Lectures in Business and Organization* (London: Management Publications Trust).

Francis, R. (2013) *Report of the Mid Staffordshire NHS Foundation Trust Public Inquiry Executive summary* (London: The Stationery Office).

Gioia, D. A., K. G. Corley and A. L. Hamilton (2012) 'Seeking Qualitative Rigor in Inductive Research: Notes on the Gioia Methodology', *Organizational Research Methods*, 16(1): 15–31.

Gilligan, C. (1982) *In a Different Voice: Psychological Theory and Women's Development* (Cambridge, MA, and London: Harvard University Press).

Grant, A. M. and S. V. Patil (2012) 'Challenging the Norm of Self-interest: Minority Influence and Transitions to Helping Norms in Work Units', *Academy of Management Review*, 37(4): 547–68.

Gross, J. J. and R. A. Thompson (2007) 'Emotion Regulation: Conceptual Foundations', in J. Gross (ed.) *Handbook of Emotion Regulation* (New York: The Guilford Press), 3–24.

Guy, M. E. (2003) 'Ties That Bind: The Link between Public Administration and Political Science', *Journal of Politics*, 65(3), 641–55.

Guy, M. E., M. A. Newman and S. Mastracci (2008) *Emotional Labour: Putting the Service in Public Service* (Armonk, NY: M.E. Sharpe).

Hsieh, C.-W., K. Yang and K.-J. Fu (2012) 'Motivational Bases and Emotional Labour: Assessing the Impact of Public Service Motivation', *Public Administration Review*, 72(2): 241–51.

Lawrence, T. B. and S. Maitlis (2012) 'Care and Possibility: Enacting an Ethic of Care through Narrative Practice', *Academy of Management Review*, 37(4): 641–63.

Lilius, J. M. (2012) 'Recovery at Work: Understanding the Restorative Side of Depleting Client Interactions', *Academy of Management Review*, 37(4): 569–88.

Madden, L. T., D. Duchon, T. M. Madden and D. A. Plowman (2012) 'Emergent Organizational Capacity for Compassion', *Academy of Management Review*, 37(4): 689–708.

Mannion, R. (2014) 'Enabling Compassionate Healthcare: Perils, Prospects, and Perspectives', *International Journal of Health Policy and Management*, 2(1): 1–3.

Mastracci, S., M. E. Guy and M. A. Newman (2012) *Working on the Razor's Edge: Emotional Labour in Crisis Response* (Armonk, NY: M.E. Sharpe).

Mastracci, S., M. A. Newman and M. E. Guy (2006) 'Appraising Emotion Work: Determining Whether Emotional Labor Is Valued in Government Jobs', *American Review of Public Administration*, 36, 123–38.

Pugh, S. D., M. Groth and T. Hennig-Thurau (2011) 'Willing and Able to Fake Emotions: A Closer Examination of the Link between Emotional Dissonance and Employee Well-Being', *Journal of Applied Psychology*, 96(2): 377–90.

Richards, J. M. and J. J. Gross (1999) 'Composure at Any Cost? The Cognitive Consequences of Emotion Suppression', *Personality and Social Psychology Bulletin*, 25(8): 1033–44.

Rynes, S. L., J. M. Bartunek, J. E. Dutton and J. D. Margolis (2012) 'Care and Compassion through an Organizational Lens: Opening up New Possibilities', *Academy of Management Review*, 37(4): 503–23.

Sawbridge, Y. (2016) 'The emotional Labour of Nursing', *Compassion in Nursing: Theory, Evidence, and Practice* (Chapter 8) (London: Palgrave).

Sheppes, G. and J. J. Gross (2011) 'Is Timing Everything? Temporal Considerations in Emotion Regulation', *Personality and Social Psychology Review*, 15(4): 319–31.

Stivers, C. M. (2000) *Bureau Men Settlement Women* (Lawrence, KS: University of Kansas Press).

Stivers, C. M. (2009) 'A Civic Machinery for Democratic Expression: Jane Addams and Public Administration'. In M. Fischer, C. Nackenoff and W. Chmielewski (eds) (2009/1902) *Jane Addams and the Practice of Democracy* (Urbana and Chicago: University of Illinois Press), pp. 87–97.

Taylor, F. W. (1911) *The Principles of Scientific Management* (New York: The Norton Library).

Waldo, D. (1948) *The Administrative State* (New York: Ronald Press).

Weber, M. (1948) *Max Weber: Essays in Sociology* (Abingdon: Routledge).

Yanow, D. and P. Schwartz-Shea (2006) *Interpretation and Method: Empirical Research Methods and the Interpretive Turn* (Armonk, NY: M.E. Sharpe).

Conclusion: What Next for Compassion in Nursing?

Alistair Hewison and Yvonne Sawbridge

Introduction

The aim of this book was to explore compassion, examine its complex nature and stimulate debate about how it is understood and applied in nursing. The contributors have addressed a number of conceptual and practical issues concerning compassion in the context of contemporary nursing practice and have provided a number of interesting insights. The purpose of this conclusion is to draw out the implications of these insights for nursing and healthcare more widely. It was recommended in a recent review that compassionate healthcare practice be situated in an overall framework of compassionate care design, incorporating actions at policy, organisational, individual and educational levels, because it is not solely about the individual performance of nurses (Crawford et al., 2014). Although blaming individuals may be cathartic, it does little to improve the overall system of care. In this concluding chapter, the intention is to identify the main macro, meso and micro issues that require attention if compassionate care is to be provided in healthcare organisations (see Figure 12.1). Consideration of the macro, meso and micro dimensions of an issue or initiative has been used in quality improvement programmes (Godfrey et al., 2008), service integration (Curry and Ham, 2010) and policy analysis (Caldwell and Mays, 2012) to provide a structure for addressing or researching complex issues. This approach is also useful in highlighting the areas that need consideration and action if compassionate care is to be provided and serves as the framework for the conclusion. This is not to suggest the issues are unconnected, because clearly policy influences practice, and action taken at a macro level has implications for the meso and micro levels. Rather, it is to provide a means of discussing the complex mix of issues in a logical way. It is also important to note that it is not possible to address every issue in detail, and so a number of key areas have been selected on the basis that they require further action or are likely to be subject to further change.

Macro – national policy and system level

Meso – regional, organisational, hospital level

Micro – ward, department, team, unit, individual level

Figure 12.1 The macro, meso and micro levels of analysis.

Macro-level Issues

There has been a considerable amount of activity with regard to national policy (see Chapter 1). This has continued, and in the review of *Compassion in Practice* (NHS England/Nursing Directorate, 2014) it is argued, 'The vision set out two years ago in the strategy for nurses, midwives and care staff is delivering tangible improvements through the implementation of clear actions within each of the six Action Areas' (see Figure 12.2) (Cummings, 2014: 2). The report collates a number of initiatives and projects focused on addressing the 'six Cs', presenting examples in the form of case studies. It is a wide-ranging report, and with regard to the 'macro' level policy issues it makes frequent reference to the Five Year Forward View (Stevens, 2014) (see Chapter 1); public health priorities and population health; and workforce issues, including staffing, nurse education and links to the NHS Leadership Programme.

Similarly, *Hard Truths: The Journey to Putting Patients First* (DH, 2014) provides a detailed report of actions taken at a policy level to build and strengthen a culture of compassionate care. However, some uncertainty remains with respect to policy statements regarding nursing staffing levels.

1. Helping people to stay independent, maximising well-being and improving health outcomes

2. Working with people to provide a positive experience of care

3. Delivering high-quality care measuring impact

4. Building and strengthening leadership

5. Ensuring we have the right staff with the right skills in the right place

6. Supporting positive staff experience

Figure 12.2 Compassion in practice strategy action areas.
Source: NHS England/Nursing Directorate, 2014.

Nurse Staffing

This is demonstrated in the approach taken to the development of guidance for safe staffing levels in the English NHS. The National Institute for Health and Care Excellence (NICE) published guidelines for adult inpatient wards and maternity (NICE, 2015). However, the Government suspended the development of any further guidance by this independent body, handing responsibility for this work to NHS England. The Safe Staffing Alliance (which is made up of nurse leaders who work together to collate evidence and campaign for safe staffing levels) expressed concern about this decision, maintaining that it is a serious backward step because NHS England cannot take an independent view on staffing and because the outcomes will be fragmented across its various initiatives, with no standardised approach to staffing levels, resulting in a serious risk to patient safety (www.safestaffing.org.uk/).

Furthermore, the alliance presented evidence from a range of studies (see Aiken et al., 2014; Ball et al., 2012, 2014; Rafferty et al., 2007, for example) to argue that one registered nurse to eight patients, plus a nurse in charge (during the week), is unsafe and not a satisfactory minimum staffing level. They contend that missed care occurs at one nurse to seven patients, so a lower ratio is needed (www.safestaffing.org.uk/). This is endorsed by some commentators who argue that legislation for a realistic legally binding minimum base line, attenuated for care levels and specialties, that can be flexed up (never down) should be introduced (Lilley, n.d.). Other analysts conclude that although there is a positive association between higher numbers of registered nurses working on wards and patient outcomes, there is a lack of agreement on the precise means of determining the correct level (Jones et al., 2015).

What is clear, though, is that without enough nurses on duty it is not possible to provide compassionate care and that the 'no more than one to eight' recommendation (no more than eight patients to one qualified nurse) (www.safestaffing.org.uk/) could be adopted as a minimum. There is concern, however, that it could become the 'maximum', negating the purpose of the recommendation (www.safestaffing.org.uk). Further research is required to provide more clarity in this area and to inform policy. For example with regard to how the guidance needs to be applicable in different care settings. Another macro issue which is often identified as being an important element in the provision of compassionate care is nurse education.

Nurse Education

The continuing debate surrounding the association of nurse education with compassionate care was rehearsed in the Introduction and is revisited here as it is an important macro issue with regard to compassion. The poles of the debate can be summarised in the following terms: one side claims that degree-level nurse education is producing nurses who consider themselves to be too clever to care (Cavendish, 2011). The other maintains there is no objective evidence to support the anecdotal view held by some that educating nurses is linked to the 'loss' of caring from the heart of the profession (Maben and Griffiths, 2008), and that to deliver care in the complex milieu of contemporary health services, nurses need to be highly educated (McKenna et al., 2006). In a review of nurse education in England, it was found that there was no evidence that degree-level nursing reduced the quality of patient care; on the contrary, it has been demonstrated that it improves patient outcomes (Willis, 2012).

In the recent *Shape of Caring Review*, a number of key issues relating to the education and development of the registered and non-registered workforce were examined (Willis, 2015). Although it states, 'Recommendations should therefore be viewed as open suggestions, as many require detailed examination, consultation and further research before implementation' (Willis, 2015: 3), it makes 34 recommendations, organised into eight key themes (see Figure 12.3), and outlines areas for action by policymakers.

1. Enhancing the voice of patients

2. Valuing the care assistant role

3. Widening access for care assistants who wish to enter nursing

4. Developing a flexible model

5. Assuring a high-quality learning environment for registered nurses

6. Assuring high-quality on-going learning for registered nurses

7. Assuring sustainable research and innovation

8. Assuring high-quality funding and commissioning (Willis 2015)

Figure 12.3 Eight themes of the *Shape of Caring Review*.

These recommendations indicate that degree-level education is regarded as the starting point for registered nurses and that healthcare assistants should be enabled to undertake degree-level studies wherever possible to enhance the quality of the nursing workforce. The initial education and continuing development of the whole of the nursing workforce is critical to the delivery of effective, compassionate care. The review sets out a comprehensive programme of consultation, negotiation and action that must be undertaken if this aspiration is to be achieved (Willis, 2015). The outcome of this process will determine whether the potential of registered nurses and healthcare assistants to deliver high-quality compassionate care will be realised.

The overarching macro-level concern is the wider environment of care and service provision. Although the term *compassion* appears more frequently in policy discourse (for example Prime Minister David Cameron stated in 2013 that this government has put compassion ahead of bureaucratic process-driven targets [Government Speeches, 2013]), concerns remain that despite the rhetoric, healthcare in England is still focused on regulation and rules and meeting financial targets, and neglects the wider root causes of the problems (Fotaki, 2013). Similarly, as Crawford et al. (2014) conclude, reducing the threat posed by a production-line mentality, with its instrumentality and time obsession, may re-humanise healthcare (p. 3596). Attention to nurse staffing and ensuring nurse education enables nurses to advocate for and deliver compassionate care are two key macro influences that will determine the extent to which compassionate care can be provided, although they need to be embedded in a culture that places compassion at the heart of care (Mannion, 2014; Lown, 2014).

Meso-level Issues

Although sufficient staffing and the education and development of nurses are influenced by government policy, there is much that occurs at the meso, or organisational level that also has an impact on the delivery of compassionate care. For example it is now widely accepted that if staff are engaged and supported in their work, they deliver better-quality care, and patient outcomes are improved (Ham, 2014; Boorman, 2009; West et al., 2006; West and Dawson, 2011). However, ensuring staff, and in this case nurses, are engaged and supported requires attention to a number of areas at the meso level. Three important considerations have been identified (Hewison and Sawbridge, 2015), which need to be taken into account at the meso level in order to create the circumstances in which compassionate care is more likely.

➢ Recognition of the emotional impact of care on nurses.

➢ The importance of leadership (particularly emotionally intelligent leadership) in supporting staff.

➢ The need to develop context-appropriate approaches to support nurses in practice.

Recognition of the Emotional Impact of Care on Nurses

The emotional impact on nurses of the sustained provision of care, often in difficult and demanding circumstances, can be considerable (Peate, 2014; Sawbridge and Hewison, 2013; Wallbank and Preece, 2010). This was explored in Chapter 8, and the concept of emotional labour (Hochschild, 2003) was used to demonstrate the links between emotion and compassion. The purpose of Chapter 8 was to address the invisibility of emotional labour in healthcare organisations (Mastracci et al., 2012). If the emotional content of nursing work is not accounted for in the organisation of healthcare work, then the negative effects of sustained unsupported emotional labour can result in 'burnout' (Smith, 1992; Gray and Smith, 2009). This has been confirmed in a recent review where it was recommended that the importance of ensuring emotional labour should be recognised and valued, and that support and supervision are in place to enable staff to cope with the varied emotional demands of their work (Riley and Weiss, 2015). Similarly, in a survey of nursing staff well-being it was concluded that nursing staff are vulnerable to burnout, but opportunities to talk through difficult issues can help. Formal supervision, mentorship or peer support can help staff cope with the emotional experiences and demands of the nursing work environment. Furthermore, it is important that employers and nursing staff themselves recognise the impact of emotional work (RCN, 2013: 7). Acceptance that the emotional component of nursing work needs to be managed is a first step; however, putting systems in place to manage it takes considerable time, effort, energy, resources and management commitment (Sawbridge and Hewison, 2014). This requires leadership and matching of the system to the needs of the staff group concerned (see below).

The Importance of Leadership in Supporting Staff

The Francis Inquiry (2013) highlighted the need for a systematic approach to leadership and management of the service, and an NHS Leadership Academy has been established (NHS Leadership Academy, 2013), which oversees the design and delivery of leadership programmes across the NHS. This signals the emphasis given to leadership at a macro level. At the meso, or organisational, level, the provision of compassionate care is contingent on the availability of effective clinical leadership. It has been suggested that the NHS needs to move beyond the outdated model of heroic leadership to recognise the value of leadership that is shared, distributed and adaptive, and that in the new model, leaders must focus on systems of care and not just institutions, and on engaging staff and followers in delivering results (King's Fund, 2011). Nurses are ideally placed to provide the clinical leadership needed to ensure these patient care outcomes are achieved (Casey et al., 2011). In recognition of this, some organisations are changing the status of their ward leaders to 'supervisory' in order that they have the time to manage and develop their team, improve performance and thus enhance the patient experience, improving patient outcomes while also contributing to organisational priorities (RCN, 2011). Because they are not included in the numbers of staff delivering direct care, they can focus their attention on leading care and ensure staff are supported to provide compassionate care. If nurses are to assume this leadership role, then appropriate development and support are required (Casey et al., 2011; Phillips and Byrne, 2013; NHS Leadership Academy, 2013); however, clinical leadership has the potential to enhance service redesign focused on patient and service user needs (Holti and Storey, 2013).

A component of leadership that has been identified as increasingly important in enabling leaders to get the best from their teams is emotional intelligence (Goleman, 1995; Goleman, Boyatzis and MacKee, 2002). Evidence exists that emotionally intelligent leaders influence employee retention, quality of patient care, and patient outcomes (Bulmer-Smith et al., 2009). Emotionally intelligent nurse leadership is characterised by self-awareness, mastery of effective supervisory skills, highlights positive empowerment processes and helps create a favourable work climate characterised by resilience, innovation and change (Akerjordet and Severinsson, 2008). It is claimed that a generation of emotionally intelligent nurse leaders who are stable, thriving and resilient can greatly enhance and transform healthcare (Codier, 2014). If this potential is to be realised, a shift may have to occur in recruitment and selection processes such that focus is on a set of competencies people must demonstrate if they are to be able to practise with compassion in high-stress environments (Sawbridge and Needham, 2014). There are several sets of competencies for emotional intelligence (see Bharwnaey et al., 2011, for a review), and these could be incorporated in the selection process for leaders in healthcare to help ensure they have appropriate skills for managing and leading care.

Developing Models of Support for Nurses in Practice

The need to support nurses in managing the emotional demands of their work has been identified throughout this book. Chapter 8, in particular, examined the importance and challenges of implementing these models in practice at the meso level, and Chapters 7 and 10 focused on two specific models of support: Schwartz Rounds and restorative supervision. These have been introduced in a number of organisations, and there is some emerging evidence to suggest they may have promise in terms of the type of support provided and sustainability (Goodrich, 2012; Bigwood, 2013).

However, there are several other approaches, that may be better suited to different contexts. Mindfulness training, for example, is one approach that has been positively related to job satisfaction and self-reported measures of wellness (Bazarko et al., 2013; Hulsheger et al., 2013). Other interventions include training to help people understand and better manage stress (Siu et al., 2014), reflection (Horton-Deutsch, 2008) and clinical supervision (Hyrkäs et al., 2005). In addition, using action research and appreciative inquiry, Dewar and Nolan (2013) identified key components of compassionate relationship-centred care and demonstrated that a compassionate environment could be created (Dewar and Nolan, 2013). Similarly, an approach designed to create learning environments for compassionate care has been investigated (Bridges and Fuller, 2015). More recently, there has been increasing interest in applying the principles of Magnet© accreditation in England (Foster, 2015a,b) (also discussed in the introduction chapter) because of its potential to promote quality, identify excellence in the delivery of nursing services to patients and provide a mechanism for disseminating best practices in nursing services (Drenkard, 2010).

This is illustrative of the range of approaches that have been or are being developed to support nursing staff in their practice. These meso-level initiatives will require further evaluation before conclusions about their impact in terms of the delivery of compassionate care can be drawn. In the final section of this chapter, the links between such approaches and what needs to be considered at the micro level are discussed.

Micro-level Issues

An area that is attracting interest with regard to action at the micro level is self-compassion. In a recent editorial, it was observed that further research is needed: first, to examine the influence of the relationship between self-compassion and self-care in nurses; then to test its relationship to compassionate care for patients. This emerging line of inquiry in nursing practice can serve to progress the imperative of compassionate care towards a compassion that is more genuine, self-compassion (Mills et al., 2015: 792). Physical fitness is important in terms of the ability to undertake the physical work of care. The same principle has been applied to emotional labour (Mastracci et al., 2012). The greater the emotional resilience an individual possesses, the more able she or he will be to manage emotion work. This view is reflected in the availability of resources which have been produced for staff. For example, Figure 12.4 illustrates a well-being assessment tool.

NHS Employers has produced a toolkit called 'How are you feeling today?', which can help individuals assess their levels of well-being. The website also has a number of resources and tips to help people improve their well-being. A key concept is their '5 steps to well-being', which outlines the important components in keeping mentally well, and provides help and support for each of these. The five steps are as follows:

➢ Get active.

➢ Connect with others.

➢ Keep learning.

➢ Be aware of yourself and the world.

➢ Give to others.

Figure 12.4 How are you feeling today?
Source: 'How Are You Feeling NHS? Toolkit', www.nhsemployers.org/howareyoufeelingnhs.

This is intended to help staff identify how they are feeling and take time to focus on their own well-being. A similar tool, which offers a free test of resilience, can be found at www.robertsoncooper.com/iresilience/. This website also offers advice about and guidance on how to improve personal resilience. Clearly, although identifying levels of individual well-being and resilience at the micro level can be helpful, support at the macro and meso levels needs to be in place if action is to be taken to address any deficits that are identified. If such support is not available and the focus is solely on the individual, there is a risk that people are seen as the 'problem'. Although staff have a responsibility to contribute to their own well-being, the organisational structures and processes need to be in place if staff are to be adequately supported in their caring work. The use of tools, such as those noted above, can provide a link between the levels of action. They can also provide a basis for the need for nurses to recognise the importance of taking care of themselves. Many nurses find it hard to take a break or leave the ward on time, as they feel patient care will suffer if they do (Chilton, 2013). Although it may appear to be counterintuitive, the opposite is the case: by looking after themselves and each other, nurses are more likely to provide good care to patients (West and Dawson, 2011). Airlines make it clear that in an emergency you must put on your own oxygen mask before helping others with theirs, and this recommendation applies to nursing with regard to compassion.

Summary

Respect, dignity, compassion and care should be at the core of how patients and staff are treated, not only because that is the right thing to do, but because patient safety, experience and outcomes are all improved when staff are valued, empowered and supported (NHS Constitution, 2015). This statement from the NHS constitution indicates that compassion should be at the heart of nursing and healthcare. The key word here is *should*. A survey identified that 8 out of 10 nurses reported they always or sometimes felt upset or distressed because they were unable to give the care they knew they should, and in excess of 98 per cent said that the dignity of their patients and clients was important to them (RCN, 2008). It has also been demonstrated that job satisfaction derived from giving good care can act as protection against the negative aspects of emotional labour (Mastracci et al., 2012). This reinforces the underlying message of this book that the provision of compassionate care requires understanding of and action in a number of areas. In a recent editorial, it was acknowledged that any strengthening of nursing values related to compassion, promulgated by education, needs to be underpinned with a shift in organisational healthcare culture (Timmins and de Vries, 2015). The aim of this book was that the analysis of macro-, meso- and micro-level issues would provide new insights on a challenging area of nursing practice, and in the conclusion the need for further research has been identified. However, what is also required is sustained and focused action. In the two-year review of the Nursing Directorate's *Compassion in Practice Strategy* (NHS England/Nursing Directorate, 2014), the chief nurse stated:

> We are now on a cusp, and the choice lies with us to either dwell on the scandals that have affected us in the past and the pressures that occupy us today, or to make a difference by working differently. We have been making progress over the past two years and have had a positive impact on patient care despite pressures. However, we can go even further by making improvements and impact with the possibilities being opened up by the Forward View. The future will bring different challenges, but also tremendous opportunities. (p. 4)

If these opportunities are to be capitalised on and compassionate nursing care is to be provided consistently, then sustained attention to the areas highlighted in this book will be needed.

Useful Resources/Websites

'How Are You Feeling NHS? Toolkit', www.nhsemployers.org/howareyoufeelingnhs.
'Free I-Resilience Report: Over 70,000 People Have Already Started Developing
  Their Resilience …', www.robertsoncooper.com/iresilience/.
'Rehumanising Healthcare', Hearts in Healthcare, http://heartsinhealthcare.com/.

References

Aiken, L., D. M. Sloane, L. Bruyneel, K. Van den Heede, P. Griffiths, M. Diomidous
  et al. (2014) 'Nurse Staffing and Education and Hospital Mortality in Nine
  European Countries: A Retrospective Observational Stud', *The Lancet*,
  383(9931): 1824–30, http://dx.doi.org/10.1016/S0140-6736(13)62631-8.
Aiken, L., D. Havens and D. Sloane (2000) 'The Magnet Nursing Services
  Recognition Program', *The American Journal of Nursing*, 100: 26–36.
Akerjordet, K. and E. Severinsson (2008) 'Emotionally Intelligent Leadership:
  A Literature Review', *Journal of Nursing Management*, 16(5): 565–77.
Ball, J. E., T. Murrells, A. M. Rafferty, E. Morrow and T. Griffiths (2014) '"Care Left
  Undone" during Nursing Shifts: Associations with Workload and Perceived
  Quality of Care', *BMJ Quality & Safety*, 23(2):116–25.
Ball, J., G. Pike, P. Griffiths, A. M. Rafferty and T. Murrells (2012) 'RN4CAST
  Nurse Survey in England', National Nursing Research Unit, www.safestaffing.
  org.uk/downloads/rn4cast-nurse-survey-in-england.
Bazarko, D., R. A. Cate, F. Azocar and M. J. Kreitzer (2013) 'The Impact of an
  Innovative Mindfulness-Based Stress Reduction Program on the Health and
  Well-being of Nurses Employed in a Corporate Setting', *Journal of Work and
  Behavioural Health*, 28(2): 107–33.
Bharwaney, G., R. Bar-On and A. MacKinlay (2011) *EQ and the Bottom Line:
  Emotional Intelligence Increases Individual Occupational Performance, Leadership
  and Organisational Productivity* (Ampthill: Ei World).
Bigwood, P. (2013) *Using Restorative Supervision to Improve Clinical Practice and
  Safeguarding Decisions* (London: Department of Health).
Boorman, S. (2009) 'The Boorman Review: Interim Report', NHS Health and
  Well-being Review, www.nhshealthandwellbeing. org/pdfs/NHS%20HWB%20
  Review%20, accessed 5 November 2015.
Bridges, J. and A. Fuller (2015) 'Creating Learning Environments for
  Compassionate Care: A Programme to Promote Compassionate Care by
  Health and Social Care Teams', *International Journal of Older People Nursing*,
  10(1): 48–58.
Bulmer-Smith, K., J. Profetto-McGrath and G. Cummings (2009) 'Emotional
  Intelligence in Nursing: An Integrative Review', *International Journal of
  Nursing Studies*, 46(12), 1624–36.

Caldwell, S.E.M. and N. Mays (2012) 'Studying Policy Implementation Using a Macro, Meso and Micro Frame Analysis: The Case of the Collaboration for Leadership in Applied Health Research & Care (CLAHRC) Programme Nationally and in North West London', *Implementation Science*, 10(32): 1–9.

Casey M., M. McNamara, G. Fealy and R. Geraghty (2011) 'Nurses' and Midwives' Clinical Leadership Development Needs: A Mixed Methods Study', *Journal of Advanced Nursing*, 67(7): 1502–13. doi: 10.1111/j.1365-2648.2010.05581.

Cavendish, C. (2011) 'More Little Greenies Would Rescue Nursing', *Times*, 29 September, www.thetimes.co.uk/tto/opinion/columnists/article3178487.ece, accessed 5 May 2012.

Codier, E. (2014) 'Making the Case for Emotionally Intelligent Leaders', *Nursing Management*, 45(1) 44–8.

Crawford P., B. Brown, M. Kavangarsnes and P. Gilbert (2014) 'The Design of Compassionate Care', *Journal of Clinical Nursing*, 23(23–24), 3589–99.

Cummings, J. (2014) 'Foreword', in *NHS England/Nursing Directorate Compassion in Practice – Two years On* (London: Department of Health), www.england.nhs.uk/wp-content/uploads/2014/12/nhs-cip-2yo.pdf, accessed 10 September 2015.

Curry, N. and C. Ham (2010) *Clinical and Service Integration – The Route to Improved Outcomes* (London: King's Fund).

Dewar, B. and M. Nolan (2013) 'Caring about Caring: Developing a Model to Implement Compassionate Relationship Centred Care in an Older People Care Setting', *International Journal of Nursing Studies*, 50(9): 1247–58.

Department of Health (DH) (2014) *Hard Truths: The Journey to Putting Patients First. Volume One of the Government Response to the Mid Staffordshire NHS Foundation Trust Public Inquiry* (London: Department of Health).

Department of Health (DH) (2015) 'NHS Constitution', www.gov.uk/government/uploads/system/uploads/attachment_data/file/473469/NHS_Constitution_large_print.pdf, accessed 9 November 2015.

Drenkard, K. (2010) 'Going for Gold: The Value of Attaining Magnet Recognition', *American Nurse Today*, 5(3), www.americannursetoday.com/going-for-the-gold-the-value-of-attaining-magnet-recognition/, accessed 9 November 2015.

Foster, S. (2015a) 'Is Magnet Hospital Status for Us?', *British Journal of Nursing*, 24(6): 335.

Foster, S. (2015b) 'Setting Our Sights on a Pathway to Practice Improvement', *British Journal of Nursing*, 24(20): 983.

Fotaki, M. (2013) 'On Compassion, Markets and Ethics of Care', Centre for Health and the Public Interest, http://chpi.org.uk/on-compassion-markets-and-ethics-of-care/, accessed 9 September 2015.

Francis, R. (2013) 'Report of the Mid Staffordshire NHS Foundation Trust Public Inquiry', www.gov.uk/government/uploads/system/uploads/attachment_data/file/279124/0947.pdf, accessed 21 August 2015.

Godfrey, M. M., G. N. Melin, S. E. Muething, P. B. Batalden and E. C. Melson (2008) 'Clinical Microsystems, Part 3: Transformation of Two Hospitals Using

Microsystem, Mesosytem and Macrosystem Strategies', *Joint Commission on Quality and Patient Safety*, 34(10): 591–603.

Goleman, D. (1995) *Emotional Intelligence* (London: Bloomsbury).

Goleman, D., R. Boyatzis and A. MacKee (2002) *The New Leaders: Transforming the Art of Leadership into the Science of Results* (London: Little Brown).

Government Speeches (2013) 'Francis Report: PM Statement on Mid Staffs Public Inquiry', 6 February, www.gov.uk/government/speeches/francis-report-pm-statement-on-mid-staffs-public-inquiry, accessed 6 February 2013.

Goodrich, J. (2012) 'Supporting Hospital Staff to Provide Compassionate Care: Do Schwartz Center Rounds Work in English Hospitals?', *Journal of the Royal Society of Medicine*, 105(3), 117–22.

Gray, B. and P. Smith, P. (2009) 'Emotional Labour and the Clinical Settings of Nursing Care: The Perspectives of Nurses in East London', *Nurse Education in Practice*, 9(4): 253–61.

Ham, C. (2014) *Staff Engagement and Empowerment in the NHS* (London: King's Fund).

Hewison, A. and Y. Sawbridge (2015) 'Organisational Support for Nurses in Acute Care Settings: A Rapid Evidence Review', *International Journal of Healthcare*, www.researchgate.net/publication/280944244_Organisational_support_for_nurses_in_acute_care_settings_a_rapid_evidence_review, accessed 21 August 2015.

Hochschild, A. R. (2003) *The Managed Heart* (Berkeley: University of California Press).

Horton-Deutsch, S. and G. Sherwood (2008) 'Reflection: An Educational Strategy to Develop Emotionally Competent Nurse Leaders', *Journal of Nursing Management*, 16(8): 946–54.

Hülsheger, U. R., H. J. Alberts, A. Feinholdt and J. W. Lang (2013) 'Benefits of Mindfulness at Work: The Role of Mindfulness in Emotion Regulation, Emotional Exhaustion, and Job Satisfaction', *Journal of Applied Psychology*, 98(2): 210–325.

Hyrkäs, K., K. Appelqvist-Schmidlechner and K. Kivimäki (2005) 'First-Line Managers' Views of the Long-Term Effects of Clinical Supervision: How Does Clinical Supervision Support and Develop Leadership in Healthcare?', *Journal of Nursing Management*, 13(3): 209–20.

Jones, A., T. Powell, S. Vougioukalou, M. Lynch and D. Kelly (2015) *Research into Nurse Staffing Levels in Wales* (Cardiff: Welsh Government Social Research), http://orca.cf.ac.uk/73771/1/Nurse%20staffing%20levels%20project%20report%20PUBL%20version.pdf, accessed 21 August 2015.

King's Fund (2011) *The Future of Leadership and Management in the NHS – No More Heroes*. Report from the King's Fund Commission on Leadership and Management in the NHS (London: King's Fund).

Lilley, R. (n.d.) 'Not Pretty', 4:1 Campaign, http://4to1.org.uk/roy-lilley-backs-mandatory-minimums-for-the-nhs/, accessed 9 September 2015.

Lown, B. A. (2014) 'Toward More Compassionate Healthcare Systems: Comment on Enabling Compassionate Healthcare: Perils, Prospects and Perspectives', *International Journal of Health Policy and Management*, 2(4): 199–200.

Maben, J. and P. Griffiths (2008) *Nurses in Society: Starting the Debate* (London: King's College).

Mannion, R. (2014) 'Enabling Compassionate Healthcare: Perils, Prospects and Perspectives', *International Journal of Health Policy and Management* 2(3): 115–17.

Mastracci, S. H., M. E. Guy and M. A. Newman (2012) *Working on the Razor's Edge: Emotional Labor in Crisis Response* (Armonk, NY: M.E. Sharpe).

McKenna, H., D. Thompson, R. Watson and I. Norman (2006) 'The Good Old Days of Nurse Training: Rose Tinted or Jaundiced View?', *International Journal of Nursing Studies*, 43(2): 135–7.

Mills, J., T. Wand and J. A. Fraser (2015) 'On Self-Compassion and Self-Care in Nursing: Selfish or Essential for Compassionate Care?', *International Journal of Nursing Studies*, 52(4): 791–3.

NHS England/Nursing Directorate (2014) *Compassion in Practice – Two Years On* (London: DH), www.england.nhs.uk/wp-content/uploads/2014/12/nhs-cip-2yo.pdf, accessed 10 September 2015.

NICE Staffing Guidance (2015), www.nice.org.uk/guidance/service-delivery--organisation-and-staffing/staffing, accessed 21 August 2015.

NHS Leadership Academy (2013) 'Healthcare Leadership Model – The Nine Dimensions of Leadership Behaviour', www.leadershipacademy.nhs.uk, accessed 30 January 2015.

Peate, I. (2014) 'Compassion Fatigue: The Toll of Emotional Labour', *British Journal of Nursing*, 23(5): 251.

Phillips, N. and G. Byrne (2013) 'Enhancing Frontline Clinical Leadership in an Acute Hospital Trust', *Journal of Clinical Nursing*, 22(17–18): 2625–35.

Rafferty, A. M., S. P. Clarke, J. Coles, J. Ball, P. James, M. McKee et al. (2007) 'Outcomes of Variation in Hospital Nurse Staffing in English Hospitals: Cross-sectional Analysis of Survey Data and Discharge Records', *International Journal of Nursing Studies*, 44(2): 175–82.

Riley, R. and M. C. Weiss (2015) 'A Qualitative Thematic Review: Emotional Labour in Healthcare Settings', *Journal of Advanced Nursing*, 72(1): 6–17. doi: 10.1111/jan.12738.

Royal College of Nursing (RCN) (2013) *Beyond Breaking Point – A Survey of RCN Members on Health, Wellbeing and Stress* (London: Royal College of Nursing).

Royal College of Nursing (2011) *Making the Business Case for Ward Sisters/Team Leaders to Be Supervisory to Practice* (London: Royal College of Nursing).

Royal College of Nursing (RCN) (2008) 'Dignity Survey', www.rcn.org.uk/newsevents/campaigns/dignity/the_rcns_dignity_survey, accessed 24 September 2015.

Sawbridge, Y. and A. Hewison (2013) 'Thinking about the Emotional Labour of Nursing – Supporting Nurses to Care', *Journal of Health Organization and Management*, 27(1): 127–33.

Sawbridge, Y. and A. Hewison (2014) 'Time to Care? An Action Research Project', www.birmingham.ac.uk/Documents/college-social-sciences/social-policy/HSMC/publications/2014/Time-To-Care-FINAL-March-2014.pdf.

Sawbridge, Y. and C. Needham (2014) 'Emotionally Qualified?', *Nursing Standard*, 29(13): 26–7.

Smith, P. (1992) *The Emotional Labour of Nursing* (Basingstoke: Macmillan Education).

Siu, O. L., C. L. Cooper and D. R. Phillips (2014) 'Intervention Studies on Enhancing Work Well-Being, Reducing Burnout, and Improving Recovery Experiences among Hong Kong Healthcare Workers and Teachers', *International Journal of Stress Management*, 21(1): 69–84.

Stevens, S. (2014) 'Five Year Forward View', www.england.nhs.uk/wp-content/uploads/2014/10/5yfv-web.pdf, accessed 30 October 2014.

Storey, J. and R. Holti (2013) *Possibilities and Pitfalls for Clinical Leadership in Improving Service Quality, Innovation and Productivity*, final report, NIHR Service Delivery and Organisation Programme (London: The Stationery Office).

Timmins, F. and de J.M.A. Vries (2015) 'Follow the Yellow Brick Road – The Compassion Deficit Debate Where to From Here?', *Journal of Clinical Nursing*, 24(1): 2689–94.

Wallbank, S. and E. Preece (2010) 'Evaluation of Clinical Supervision Given to Health Visitor and School Nurse Leadership Participants'. NHS West Midlands and Worcester University.

West, M. and J. Dawson (2011) 'NHS Staff Management and Health Service Quality', www.gov.uk/government/uploads/system/uploads/attachment_data/file/215454/dh_129658.pdf, accessed 5 November 2015.

West, M. A., J. P. Guthrie, J. F. Dawson, C. S. Borrill and M. Carter (2006) 'Reducing Patient Mortality in Hospitals: The Role Of Human Resource Management', *Journal of Organizational Behavior*, 27(7): 983–1002.

Willis, P. (Chair) (2012) *Quality with Compassion: The Future of Nurse Education* (London: Royal College of Nursing).

Willis, P. (2015) Raising the Bar *Shape of Caring: A Review of the Future Education and Training of Registered Nurses and Care Assistants* (London: Health Education England).

Index